STUDENT NOTES

Fractures and Orthopaedics

David F. Paton
MB FRCS FRCSE
Consultant Orthopaedic Surgeon
Whittington Hospital and
Royal Northern Hospital;
Honorary Consultant Orthopaedic Surgeon
The Italian Hospital;
Formerly, Professor of Orthopaedic Surgery
University of Cape Town

CHURCHILL LIVINGSTONE
EDINBURGH LONDON MELBOURNE AND NEW YORK 1988

CHURCHILL LIVINGSTONE
Medical Division of Longman Group UK Limited

Distributed in the United States of America by Churchill
Livingstone Inc., 1560 Broadway, New York, N.Y.
10036, and by associated companies, branches and rep-
resentatives throughout the world.

First published 1988
Reprinted 1989
Parts I and II previously published by Churchill
Livingstone as *Notes on Fractures* by the same author.

ISBN 0-443-03754-X

British Library Cataloguing in Publication Data

Paton, David F.
 Fractures and orthopaedics.
 1. Fractures.
 I. Title
 617'.15   RD101

Library of Congress Cataloging-in-Publication Data

Paton, David F.
 Fractures and orthopaedics.

 Includes index.
 1. Fractures. 2. Orthopedia. I. Title.
[DNLM: 1. Bone and Bones—surgery. 2. Bone Disease—
therapy. 3. Fractures. 4. Orthopedics. WE 180 P312f]
RD101.P36 1988   617'.15   87-15862

Produced by Longman Singapore Publishers Pte Ltd
Printed in Singapore.

To my daughter Fiona

Acknowledgements

I wish to thank Mr Martin Lowy for reading through the text and offering many helpful suggestions, the surgeons who taught me and finally the students whose interest stimulated me to write this book.

Preface

This book is to teach medical students all they need to know about fractures and orthopaedics. It is also hoped that the book will prove of use to nurses, physiotherapists and students of other paramedical disciplines.

Recognizing that medical students have a vast amount of factual knowledge to digest, the author has developed a system of teaching which demands the least possible learning by rote.

In the section devoted to fractures, the student *must* learn the 'general principles of fracture treatment' (Part I). After that he or she will be asked to memorize only that information which is peculiar to or particular to the individual fracture under discussion. It will be taken for granted that the student will apply the general principles already learned.

The section on orthopaedics has been written to show how closely and how logically the clinical presentation of any condition follows the pathology. An understanding of the pathology often makes it quite unnecessary to memorize lists of clinical findings—they can be logically deduced in most cases. Much of orthopaedics can be covered in this manner by a series of pathology-based topics.

However, and unfortunately, orthopaedics is blessed or cursed with a miscellany of conditions which do not conveniently fit into general topics. Previous textbooks have attempted to overcome this difficulty by teaching the subject on a regional (anatomical) basis. This results in repetition as similar pathology may be mentioned under sections on spine, pelvis, shoulder, arm, hip etc. This seems to the author unneccesary and illogical. Having learned, for example, how acute pyogenic osteitis presents, the student can reasonably be expected to apply this presentation to various parts of the anatomy. Any notable exceptions to these rules receive special mention in the book.

Such miscellany as does not fit into general topics has, the author regrets, to be dealt with regionally. The author apologises for this but pleads in mitigation that this small book should be comprehensive enough within its few pages to prepare medical students for final examinations, to advise junior doctors on the principles of orthopaedic surgery and medicine, and to assist in the training of nurses, physiotherapists and other paramedical staff.

The author makes no apology for directing this book towards the requirements of examiners as well as the more important area of clinical practice. The book is based on the system of teaching fractures and orthopaedics which the author has used over many years.

London, 1988   D.F.P.

Contents

Part I
General principles of fracture treatment

Classification

A fracture indicates a complete or partial break in the continuity of a bone. Fractures may be classified in three ways:

I. ACCORDING TO THE CAUSATION OF THE FRACTURE

A. Traumatic fractures
The vast majority of fractures are caused by trauma. The injury may be caused by direct violence, indirect violence or by the violence of muscular pull. Examples of these are:

Direct violence e.g. the ulna is fractured when the arm is put up to ward off a blow with a stick.

Indirect violence e.g. a fall on the outstretched hand may fracture the head of the radius or the clavicle. Here the force is transmitted up the arm.

Muscular pull e.g. the patella may be fractured by a sudden violent contraction of the quadriceps muscle.

B. Stress or fatigue fractures
In these fractures the bone is fatigued by repetitive stress in much the same way as metal fatigues in aircraft e.g. stress fracture of the fibula in athletes.

C. Pathological fractures
A pathological fracture is one in which the fracture occurs through a bone already weakened by underlying disease. Not surprisingly the trauma may be quite trivial or the fracture occur spontaneously. Indeed, this fact may lead the clinician to suspect that the fracture is pathological.

Causes of pathological fractures: General
                                     Local

Generalized disease of skeleton
  1. Disseminated tumours and myelomatosis

2. Osteoporosis — prolonged immobility
                    — old age
                    — hormonal factors
3. Metabolic conditions — involving metabolism of
   calcium, phosphorus and vitamin D. Rickets and
   osteomalacia may result from dietary deficiencies,
   malabsorbtion from the intestine or loss of salts from
   renal tubular disease.
4. Adrenal hypercorticalism or excessive steroid therapy.

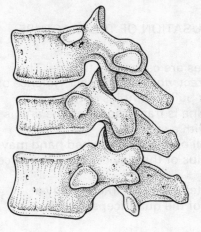

Vertebral body crush fracture
typical of metastatic bone
disease or osteoporosis

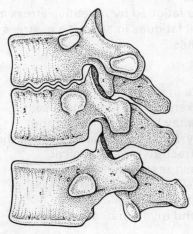

Compare this with the destruction
of disc space and adjacent bone
which is typical of infection

Fig. 1

5. Hyperparathyroidism.
6. Paget's disease.
7. Neuropathic conditions — syphilis
                                 — syringomyelia
8. Osteogenesis imperfecta.

Local disease of bone
1. Metastases in bone from malignant tumours elsewhere. Typically these arise from carcinomata of *breast, prostate, thyroid, kidney* and *bronchus.*
2. Malignant primary bone tumours.
3. Benign primary bone tumours.
4. Hyperaemia and infective decalcification, e.g. osteitis.
5. Miscellaneous local conditions:
   — simple bone cyst
   — fibrous dysplasia
   — eosinophilic granuloma
   — bone atrophy e.g. polio or meningomyelocoele
   — X-radiation of bone
   — hyatid disease

II. ACCORDING TO THEIR RELATION TO SURROUNDING TISSUES

A. **Simple fractures**
The overlying skin is healthy and closed.

B. **Compound fractures**
The skin has been breached and the fracture site itself exposed to contamination. Note that fractures may also become compound by communication with unsterile body cavities, e.g. air sinuses, mouth etc.

C. **Complicated fractures**
In association with the fracture other important structures have been damaged e.g. nerves, vessels, viscera or joints.

III. ACCORDING TO THE PATTERN OF THE FRACTURE

A. **Complete fractures**
The bone is completely divided into two separate fragments. The fracture line itself may be transverse, oblique or spiral.

Often this pattern gives evidence of the nature of the
violence and also of the stability of the fracture.

B. **Incomplete fractures**
 1. In children — the bones have an elasticity which permits
    them to crack and buckle within the periosteal sheath.
    These are Greenstick fractures.
 2. In adults — incomplete fractures are found as the result
    of impaction. Here the bone fragments have been
    jammed into each other and are thus stable.

C. **Comminuted fractures**
There are more than two fragments.

D. **Compression or crush fractures**
These usually occur in cancellous bone.

Displacement of fragments

The following forces tend to displace a complete fracture: Original violence, muscle pull and gravity. Displacement is described by the movement of the distal fragment on the proximal. Four such displacements are important:

1. *Of alignment*: This refers to a disturbance of the normal longitudinal axis of the bone so as to alter the line through which stress is carried. Restoration of this axis to

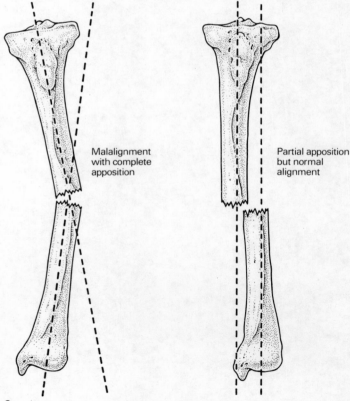

Malalignment with complete apposition

Partial apposition but normal alignment

Fig. 2

normal is important for the continued health of adjacent joints.

2. *Of length:* Shortening can be produced by overlapping of fragments and lengthening by distraction of fragments.

3. *Of apposition*: This refers to the relationship between the bone ends. Ideally this should be complete but union will usually occur even if apposition is incomplete. Note that partial apposition may still permit normal alignment provided that the longitudinal axis of each fragment is parallel to that of the other.

4. *Of rotation:* The distal fragment may rotate on the proximal, about the longitudinal axis of the bone. This displacement should be looked for clinically as it is not easy to see on radiographs.

The diagnosis of a fracture

I. HISTORY

There is a history of trauma. Enquire about the nature of the injury as this information may suggest the type of fracture. If trauma is trivial or absent, consider the possibility of a pathological fracture.

Always enquire about any other injuries. Never forget the possibility of *associated injuries*.

Take a brief general history with attention to establishing the fitness of the patient for anaesthesia. The following points will avoid embarrassing the anaesthetist:

? State of cardiovascular and respiratory systems.

? Presence of diabetes.

? Patient on steroid therapy.

? Patient taking any other drugs or allergic to any drugs.

? Time of last food or drink.

II. EXAMINATION

A. Pain and tenderness are usually present, both over the fracture and on moving the part.

B. Swelling and bruising.

C. Deformity.

D. Abnormal mobility, i.e. movements where no joint exists.

E. Absence of transmitted movements.

F. Loss of function.

G. Crepitus. This may be found incidentally, but should not be deliberately elicited.

H. Discrepancies in length of limbs.

I. A *routine examination to exclude associated injuries*.

J. A *routine examination to exclude complications of fracture*.

A search should be made for wounds indicating that the fracture is compound. The nerves supplying the part concerned should be tested. The blood supply of the limb must be examined. Observe the peripheral pulses, colour of skin, temperature of skin, capillary return etc.

NOTE: When making notes about the examination, it is wise for medicolegal reasons to write down that other injuries and complications have been excluded.

III. RADIOGRAPHIC EXAMINATION

An X-ray should be taken whenever there is the possibility of a fracture. Two films at right angles to each other are usually taken and you should ask for these.

In certain circumstances extra films are of value. Oblique views and comparison films of the normal limb may then be requested, e.g. in suspected fractures of the elbow in children the epiphyses may give rise to diagnostic difficulties. A comparison film of the normal side is of great help.

Radiographs are also used to confirm that reduction has been achieved and subsequently to follow the progress of union.

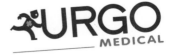

The healing of fractures

The healing of fractures is in five main stages:

1. **Haematoma formation**

2. **Organization of haematoma**
Within hours of this injury fibroblasts from adjacent tissues begin to enter the haematoma and within a few days capillary buds grow into it. The result is the gradual organization of the haematoma to granulation tissue.

3. **Callus formation**
The fibroblasts in the granulation tissue show metaplasia and change into collagenoblasts, chondroblasts and later to osteoblasts. Osteoblasts from adjacent healthy bone also participate. Bone is laid down in a haphazard fashion around collagen fibres and islets of cartilage. This is called WOVEN BONE. The callus causes the fracture to become firm and may be felt as a mass. It is visible on a radiograph.

4. **Consolidation by mature bone**
The woven bone is replaced by lamellar bone.

5. **Remodelling**
Excess callus is removed and the bone resumes a normal or near normal shape. The medullary canal is recanalized. Children have great powers of remodelling and may correct deformities and even discrepancies of length after a fracture.

TIME NECESSARY FOR UNION

This varies quite widely and differs between one bone and another. However, the following rule of thumb is helpful:
— Cortical bone requires 3 months to heal in adults.
— Cancellous bone requires 6 weeks to heal in adults.
— Children require about half as long as adults.

Principles of fracture treatment

FIRST AID

In principle this consists of measures to limit pain and to prevent further damage by excessive movement of the fragments. Elaborate splintage may cause pain and waste time if the patient does not have far to travel to hospital. Such measures as a sling for upper limb fractures and bandaging to the normal leg in lower limb fractures are simple and effective. Prevent bystanders from giving the patient, 'a nice cup of tea' as he may require an anaesthetic.

Compound fractures should be covered with the cleanest material available. Otherwise treatment is as above.

TREATMENT OF SHOCK

It is important to know that the fracture of a large bone may be associated with considerable blood loss, e.g. 1litre — 1.5 litre of blood may frequently be lost around a fractured femur. Hence in cases with multiple fractures oligaemic shock may be present. Neurogenic shock due to pain may be superadded. Such cases require urgent transfusion with blood or plasma volume expanders.

Beware of sending a patient off to the X-ray department without an intravenous infusion as he may become shocked while not under observation. It is important to add, that adequate doses of analgesics should be given early provided that there are no contraindications.

PRELIMINARY ASSESSMENT

Careful examination is necessary to establish a baseline for subsequent observations. The facts of this examination must then be recorded. It must be emphasised again that *associated injuries* and *complications* of the fracture must be sought and excluded.

AIMS OF TREATMENT OF FRACTURE ITSELF (Fig. 3)

1. *Reduction.* This means the restoration of the displaced fragments to their anatomical position.
2. *Immobilization or fixation.* This means retention of the fragments in the reduced position until union.
3. *Achievement of union.*
4. *Restoration of function.*

Reduction

The decision as to whether a fracture requires reduction or not is one of the main arts of fracture treatment. In general, it may be said that in cases where the displacement is very slight, or where function of the limb may be restored to normal without anatomical reduction, or in children who have greater powers of remodelling, small displacements may be accepted. In general, imperfect alignment is less acceptable than imperfect apposition. It must be repeated that considerable experience is required in these decisions. A fracture that requires manipulation requires an anaesthetic. Local and regional anaesthetics have their place, but a general anaesthetic is desirable in any major fracture as it produces muscle relaxation.

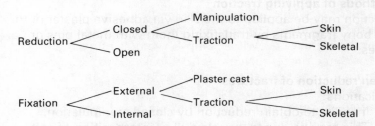

Fig. 3 Summary of methods of fracture treatment

Methods of reduction

1. Manipulative reduction of the fracture with external fixation in a plaster cast.
2. Manipulative reduction and fixation by skin or skeletal traction.
3. Reduction by mechanical traction.
4. Mechanical reduction of the fracture, controlling the fragments and fixing them by skeletal transfixation.

5. Open reduction of the fracture usually with internal fixation, but sometimes with external splintage.

Plaster technique
Students should ensure that they have practised the art of plaster bandaging.

It is advisable always to plaster over a layer of plaster wool.

If considerable swelling is present it may be preferable to use a plaster slab only at first and complete this to a full plaster at a later date.

The position of the fragments should be checked by X–ray in the plaster.

Instructions should be given to outpatients to report any tightness or signs of vascular impairment in the limb.

Every plaster should be checked on the following day.

Indications for traction
1. Where powerful muscles tend to cause shortening or angulation of the fracture, e.g. fracture of femur.
2. Extremely unstable fractures, e.g. oblique fractures which tend to shorten.

Methods of applying traction
Traction may be applied to the skin via adhesive plaster or to the bony fragments by transfixing them with metal pins or wires.

Open reduction of fractures
Indications:
1. Inability to obtain reduction by closed manipulation. This may be due to muscle pull or interposition of soft tissues. Intra-articular fractures may require this to restore articular surfaces.
2. Inability to maintain reduction due to instability of fractures. The fracture may slip after a perfect initial reduction.
3. Some surgeons believe that rigid internal fixation by special plates etc. ensure the best chance of early union. However, if fixation is inadequate, union may, in fact, be delayed by open reduction.
4. Internal fixation permits early mobilization of adjacent

joints, but weight bearing must be delayed until union is well advanced.

The great danger of open reduction is that it converts a simple fracture into a compound fracture and ensuing infection may prove very difficult to eradicate. This risk has often to be taken to ensure a good result.

Optimum time for open reduction
If early reduction is desirable, then the sooner the better is the axiom. However, certain fractures are not disadvantaged if open reduction is delayed for 10 to 14 days, e.g. fracture of the femur.

Methods of internal fixation (Fig. 4)

1. *Suturing with wire or other suture*

2. *Screwing of fracture with stainless steel or alloy screws*

3. *Plating of fracture*
The fracture is splinted internally by use of a plate fastened to both fragments by screws. Recent improvements in design of instrumentation and internal fixation devices have allowed 'rigid' internal fixation. Compression of the bone ends can be added further to improve fixation. Fractures treated by these methods heal well without forming much external callus. There is some doubt whether 'rigid' fixation is always advantageous and very recently 'semi-rigid' plates have been introduced to encourage external callus formation. Occasionally 'double' plating with plates at right angles to each other may be needed for difficult fractures.

4. *Intramedullary nailing*
The passage of an intramedullary nail along a fractured tubular bone can achieve fixation which is mechanically very strong. By careful attention to reaming of the canal quite large nails may be introduced to produce the best possible fixation.

5. *External fixation devices*
Here the fragments are transfixed by pins which are assembled and held in an external fixation device to give very effective immobilisation of the fragments. By careful adjustment of the pins before they are clamped into the

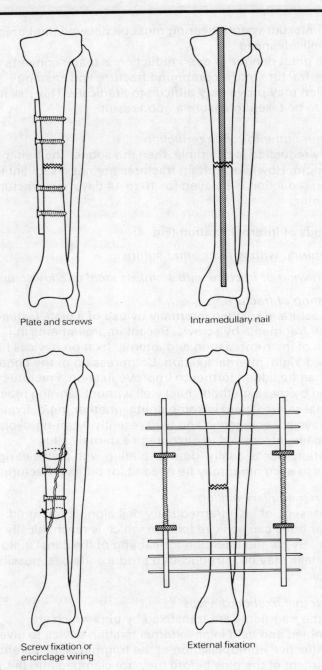

Plate and screws

Intramedullary nail

Screw fixation or
encirclage wiring

External fixation

Fig. 4

fixator, very awkward and comminuted fractures can be reduced and held.

This technique is of special advantage when there is much damage to skin and soft tissues. The fracture can be held while the surgeon has access to the damaged tissues for dressings, skin grafting etc.

Recent improvements in the design and versatility of fixators and the shape of the pins have permitted very efficient fixation of difficult fractures without the loosening and pin track infection which used to bedevil this method.

Restoration of function

The restoration of function of the injured part and the rehabilitation of the patient as a whole is of the greatest importance in the management of fractures. Less dramatic than early surgical procedures, it tends to be forgotten.

Preventative measures

Oedema and subsequent stiffness are closely linked, especially in injuries to the wrist and hand. Where considerable oedema is present, admission to hospital for elevation of the part is desirable. In less severe cases a sling suffices. Similarly, in injuries to the leg, elevation of the part reduces swelling.

All outpatients with fractures must be given specific advice to exercise as much of the injured limb as is accessible, e.g. in a case of Colles fracture the patient must be taught to exercise fingers, elbow and shoulder.

It is not necessary to refer every outpatient for physiotherapy. However, those cases with oedema and early stiffness must be looked for and referred for treatment. Inpatients can usually be supervised, both by the clinician and physiotherapist, but nevertheless advice to exercise on their own should be given.

Active use

As much use of the injured part must be encouraged as is compatible with successful treatment of the fracture.

Active exercises and physiotherapy

Even when a limb is splinted, the muscles must be actively exercised. Static contractions are encouraged. As soon as rigid splinting is no longer essential, gradual movement of the joints must be encouraged.

Active movements are always preferable to passive stretching. In the elbow, passive stretching can lead to myositis ossificans.

When the fracture is soundly united, treatment is intensified until the part is returned to normal, or near normal.

Return to normal living and employment

The return of the patient to normal daily activities including employment must be the aim of the clinician. The patient may need firm encouragement to return to work. Help may be necessary from employers, occupational therapists, social workers and resettlement officers. If there appears to be any inexplicable delay in return to work, tactful enquiries about litigation may reveal the cause. In these cases the advice of the resettlement or rehabilitation units is often a great help.

Treatment of compound fractures

The object of treatment of a compound fracture is to try to prevent the contaminated wound from becoming infected. Infection leads to osteomyelitis, which may be difficult to eradicate. It may be discussed under the following headings:

1. *First Aid*
(vide supra)

2. *Resuscitation*
In compound fractures blood loss may be external as well as internal but otherwise the basic principles of resuscitation as previously discussed apply.

3. *Preliminary assessment*
(vide supra).

4. *Antibacterial therapy*
Antibiotics should be given as soon as the diagnosis is made. Ideally large doses of suitable antibiotics should be given by intramuscular injection e.g. Benzyl penicillin 1 mega unit six hourly plus flucloxacillin 500 mg six hourly should be adequate in most cases. If the wound is grossly

contaminated, gentamycin should be added with the usual attention to renal function and serum levels where these investigations are available. This treatment should be continued until the clinician is certain that the wound is not infected. Antitetanus precautions must be taken. Human antiserum is now available and should be used in patients who are not presently immunized. Otherwise a tetanus toxoid booster-dose may be given. Adequate antibiotic therapy plus surgical cleansing should protect adequately against gas gangrene.

5. *Treatment of wound and of fracture*
Compound fractures require early treatment and operation should not be delayed. The object of treatment is to cleanse the wound, remove all contaminating material and to excise the dead and devitalized tissue. The extent of the wound determines the extent of the surgery. A simple puncture wound may need no more than cleansing and suturing. Any wound where there is a possibility of contamination requires exploration and a surgical toilet.

If necessary, the wound is enlarged. A narrow strip of skin at the margin of the wound, together with any bruised or crushed tags, is excised. All crushed tissue is exposed and the fascia overlying it is incised and laid open.

The wound is thoroughly cleansed with saline or detergent solution and foreign material carefully removed. The emphasis should be on cleansing, rather than excision, of tissue. However, any crushed or devitalized muscle should be excised to prevent infection by gas gangrene organisms.

Small pieces of bone unattached to soft tissue may be picked out, but generally bone fragments should be left.

Damage to major blood vessels is dealt with at the time, but nerves are left for later suture. The ends of severed nerves should be tacked lightly together to facilitate identification later and to prevent retraction.

Skin closure by primary suture, or skin grafting should be attempted with the following exceptions. If contamination has been gross, or if the injury is older than 12 hours, it must be regarded as infected and left open. Packing with sterile gauze encourages drainage. Delayed wound closure may be necessary in such cases.

The matter of internal fixation in compound fractures arouses controversy. In the main, it is thought to be inadvisable to fix a compound fracture internally as the hazard of infection is increased. An exception to this is the case where soft tissue damage is so gross that fixation of the fracture is essential for the survival of the soft tissue. In cases needing arterial repair, fixation is advisable.

Internal fixation may, of course, be performed at a later date when the skin is healed and no evidence of infection exists. The use of external fixation devices may permit awkward compound fractures to be fixed even in the presence of severe soft tissue damage.

6. *After care of compound fracture*
The wound is inspected through a window in the plaster if necessary at about 10 to 14 days. If clean and healed the sutures are removed and further treatment is as for simple fracture. If the wound is infected then treatment is as for osteomyelitis, but union must be the aim of treatment.

The complications of fractures

1. The fracture may be complicated by *associated injuries*.
2. The fracture may be complicated by injuries to nerves, vessels, viscera, joints or ligaments.
3. Complications of fracture itself.

NERVE INJURIES

Primary nerve injuries are caused at the time of the fracture by *contusion*, *stretching* or *division* of the nerve. The term 'neuropraxia' is used to describe a minor injury in which a physiological block is caused and recovery may be expected in a few weeks. The term 'axonotomesis' refers to an injury which damages axons sufficiently to cause peripheral degeneration, but leaves the architecture of the axon tubes undamaged. The axon regenerates at the rate of about 1 mm per day and recovery may thus take months. The term 'neurotomesis' refers to destruction of the whole nerve and subsequent fibrosis defeats efforts at regeneration. Normally excision of the damaged section and suture is required before there can be a chance of recovery in a case of neurotomesis.

In closed fractures, it may be assumed that the lesion is recoverable and treatment is conservative. Physiotherapy to maintain movements in the paralysed joints and splintage to prevent overstretching of the paralysed muscles by functioning antagonist muscles or gravity is necessary.

If recovery does not occur in the expected time exploration of the nerve is advisable.

In open fractures it is usually assumed that the nerve has been divided and exploration and suture are usually performed about four weeks after the injury. If the nerve is found to be in continuity it is left and the wound closed.

Nerves may also be involved later in callus causing a 'secondary nerve injury'.

INJURIES TO BLOOD VESSELS

The vessel may be contused, lacerated or severed. Superadded *thrombosis* or *spasm* exacerbate the ischaemia. Arterial spasm may be extensive even when the actual segment traumatised is quite small and the damage relatively minor.

Further diminution of the blood supply to the extremity may be caused by *tension* within the fascial sheath due to oedema and haemorrhage.

Certain fractures are prone to vascular injuries, particularly supracondylar fractures of humerus and femur. An important example of this is the condition of Volkmann's ischaemic contracture of the forearm. Typically this results from injuries in the region of the elbow joint in children, the most common being the supracondylar fracture. The contracture is the late result of fibrosis of the deep muscles of the forearm which have undergone ischaemic necrosis. Indications of ischaemia after injury are:

A. Excessive pain.
B. Absent radial pulse.
C. Pallor or duskiness of the fingers.
D. Poor capillary return.
E. Inability to extend passively the fingers.

The condition is not unknown in the deep muscles of the calf after tibial fractures, but is less often recognized.

Treatment is an urgent matter and depends upon:

1. If the fracture is as yet unreduced, early reduction is essential.
2. If the fracture has been reduced, all constricting bandages, plasters etc. must be removed and excessive flexion of the elbow relaxed.
3. If this does not help, the lesion must be explored. Sometimes division of the fascia alone relieves tension and spasm. Hanging the arm over the side of the table for 10–15 minutes often restores circulation once the fascia has been divided. Occasionally the artery itself has to be exposed. Spasm may then be relieved by stroking the vessel or bathing it in paraverine solution.

Rarely, excision of the damaged segment is required with or without repair.

Cooling of the affected limb helps to reduce metabolic demands.

THE COMPARTMENTAL SYNDROME

In certain fascial compartments muscle ischaemia can arise without there being a major arterial injury. Swelling of muscle occurs and the intracompartmental pressure rises. When the pressure exceeds diastolic pressure then ischaemia commences as a result of small vessel occlusion. Note, however that major vessels passing through the compartment may still transmit pulsation distally until the intracompartmental pressure reaches the systolic blood pressure.

Intracompartmental pressure may arise from a variety of causes. Obviously trauma must be the most important but the condition has been described even as a result of muscle swelling after heavy exercise.

This mechanism plays an important role in the forearm ischaemia described above. Other compartments where this occurs lie in the deep flexors of the calf, the anterior tibial compartment and the peroneal compartment.

It is very important that surgeons should be aware of the existence of compartmental syndrome as this information emphasises the importance of early fasciotomy which is the only way in which this particular source of muscle ischaemia can be relieved.

COMPLICATIONS OF THE FRACTURE ITSELF

1. Delayed union

This is a clinical term which refers to a fracture which does not unite within the expected average time. Treatment is expectant, but there comes a time when the clinician has to regard the delayed union as a case of non union and treat accordingly.

2. Non-union

Here the attempts at repair have come to an end. There is a typical radiological appearance. The bone ends are sclerosed. No trabeculae cross the fracture line which indeed becomes more apparent. The marrow cavity becomes closed. In extreme cases the body attempts to create a false joint or 'pseudarthrosis'.

Causes of non-union
a. Infection.
b. Poor blood supply.
c. Excessive movement at fracture site.
d. Loss of apposition of fragments, particularly distraction.
e. Corrosion of metal used to internally fix the fracture.
f. Interposition of soft tissues between the bone ends.
g. Underlying disease of bone in pathological fractures.

Treatment of non-union
The treatment is by bone grafting with or without internal fixation. Cortical bone or cancellous bone may be used. Most frequently today cancellous bone is used packed between and around the fragments. Clinical reasearch is in progress to evaluate the use of electrical stimulation of union in cases of delayed or non-union.

3. Mal-union
This term means that the fracture has united in a position of deformity. This usually indicates a failure of treatment. Interference with alignment may cause the adjacent joints to be at a mechanical disadvantage with early ensuing secondary osteoarthritis. Whether treatment is required or not depends upon the degree of deformity, age of patient, fitness for surgery and age of the fracture. If the fracture is not yet united, deformity may be corrected by manipulation or wedging of the plaster. When it is united the bone has to be refractured or divided. In general mal-union affects more seriously weight bearing joints than non weight bearing joints.

4. Joint stiffness
Intra-articular and peri-articular adhesions limit movements of the joint affected. Physiotherapy may have to be continued for long periods, e.g. up to a year, to restore function. Occasionally a gentle manipulation under anaesthesia is useful, particularly with intra-articular adhesions.
  Joint stiffness is much more likely in a joint previously abnormal than in a normal joint. Hence children often regain full movements almost immediately, whereas the aged with their osteoarthritic joints cannot tolerate prolonged immobilization without becoming stiff.

5. Pathological ossification

Post-traumatic ossification, often called 'myositis ossificans', results from ossification in a haematoma beneath periosteum and soft tissues stripped from the bone by the injury. The elbow is the joint most affected, but it is also seen in the quadriceps muscles and anterior to the ankle, occasionally.

Resting the elbow for three weeks after a severe injury, and the avoidance of passive stretchings are the best ways to avoid this.

In the established case, passive movements must be stopped and active exercise continued. If the disability is great, surgical excision of the abnormally situated bone may be performed, but only when it is 'mature'.

6. Avascular necrosis of bone

Death of part or the whole of one fragment may result from the cutting off of its blood supply by the accident. This ischaemic necrosis may result in non-union or collapse of the fragment with early osteoarthritis or disorganization of the joint. It usually occurs in sites where the fracture divides the major part of the blood supply to one fragment. The necrotic bone is unable to withstand stress and collapses, often before the process of revascularization can take place.

It may be diagnosed radiologically because the avascular fragment appears more dense on the radiograph than the adjacent bone.

The following sites are most common:

— The head of the femur.

— The proximal half of the carpal scaphoid bone.

— The body of the talus.

— The lunate bone.

There is no specific treatment in the acute stage. In the lower limb weight bearing must be avoided in the hope that healing will occur without deformity. Later surgery is often required for the disorganized joint.

Recognition that this complication can occur is of medicolegal importance.

7. **Reflex sympathetic dystrophy** (Eponym: Sudek's osteodystrophy)

This is a condition which occasionally follows sprains or fractures, e.g. Colles fracture. The cause is unknown. Some believe that it is merely severe disuse atrophy of bone, but others believe that there may be temporary abnormality of the sympathetic nervous supply of the limb.

The hand or foot becomes painful, swollen and stiff. It has a reddened, smooth glossy and swollen appearance. Radiographs show a typical patchy osteoporosis.

Treatment requires prolonged, sympathetic but firm physiotherapy. On the whole the prognosis is good.

8. **Osteoarthritis**

This condition may result from an irregularity of the joint surface in any fracture entering a joint, or as a result of the mechanical wear and tear occasioned by functioning adjacent to a malaligned fracture. In the latter case the osteoarthritis may not set in for many years.

9. **Fat embolism**

This condition is a rare complication of major long bone fractures. It is probably more common than is realized, as minor cases are not diagnosed.

Globules of fat from the fracture site enter the venous system and pass through the lungs to the systemic circulation. The fat can cause embolic occlusion of tiny vessels, but it is probable that there is an additional toxic effect as yet not understood. Where the fat comes from is still a matter for controversy.

The clinical features vary slightly as the main effect may be on the brain or on the lungs. They may appear within a few hours to a few days after the fracture.

The patient, who was previously well, may become drowsy and irritable. The pulse and temperature rise, sometimes in bizarre fashion. Petechiae appear on the neck, upper chest, shoulders and axillae in about 20% of cases. In the cerebral type drowsiness may lead to coma and death.

In the pulmonary type the patient becomes cyanosed and develops signs of pulmonary congestion. The PO_2 falls and this is the most useful diagnostic sign in all cases.

The urine and sputum may contain fat globules. X–rays of the chest show a 'misty' appearance in the lung fields.

There is no proven successful treatment and most cases are treated symptomatically. Oxygen therapy with ventilation if necessary may be life saving in severe cases.

10. **Iatrogenic**
a. You may get away with bad treatment of a good fracture or good treatment of a bad fracture but you will scarcely ever get away with bad treatment of a bad fracture.
b. Don't miss associated injuries or complications.
c. Don't let your plasters or splints cause oedema or pressure lesions. Remember the patient is always right if he complains of discomfort.
d. Follow all the rules all the time.

General problems in the management of injuries to elderly patients

1. The patient may be frail and be 'knocked about' by the injury and any anaesthesia or surgery. This may result in confusion and disorientation.
2. The patient may have only just been able to manage by 'tottering' about. The injury may be the last straw and make rehabilitation very difficult.
3. Elderly patients removed from a well known home environment often become confused and disorientated when moved to hospital.
4. Elderly patients tend to lie too still after injuries and are prone to the following conditions:
   — pressure sores
   — bronchopneumonia
   — urinary tract infections
   — fluid and electrolyte disturbances
   — deep vein thrombosis and pulmonary embolism
5. These patients are often osteoporotic to start with and prolonged immobilization aggravates this.
6. These patients are often obese and prolonged immobilization makes them too weak to carry this weight around.
7. These patients are often weak to start with and prolonged immobilization aggravates this.
8. These patients often have pre-existing medical diseases and are generally unfit.
9. 'Disposal' is an ugly word but nevertheless disposal of these patients is often a problem. In uncaring societies the lonely aged often have nowhere to go if they are unable to return home and thus become burdens on available social services.

OSTEOPOROSIS AND OSTEOMALACIA

Elderly persons often have thinner and weaker bones and

are thus more prone to skeletal injury. In this sense such fractures may be regarded as pathological.

There are many causes for osteoporosis but the common variety affecting old people is due to the hormonal changes of later life, particularly in postmenopausal women. It is well known that oestrogen and androgen levels or a combination of the two influence osteoblastic activity. Osteoporosis is the result of failure in the production of adequate amounts of organic bone matrix, osteoid.

Histologically, osteoporotic bone shows thinning of the compacta and widening of the Haversian canals. The trabeculae of cancellous tissue are thin and often distorted by fracture. The ratio of bone mass to medullary soft tissue is greatly decreased and there are considerably fewer osteoblasts than in normal bone.

Radiologically, osteoporotic bones show greater translucency than normal. The cortices are thin and trabeculae fine and rather sparse. There may be pathological fractures such as the commonly seen compression fractures of vertebrae.

The osteoporosis of the elderly may be worsened by disuse atrophy particularly if these patients are confined to bed for a few weeks. Poor teeth or general disinterest in preparing food may result in a diet deficient in protein, calorie intake, calcium and vitamin D so that osteomalacia may add to the weakening of the osteoporotic bones.

Osteomalacia is a condition in which there is an inadequate amount of calcium or phosphorus or both for mineralization of osteoid which is formed to replace bone lost by normal catabolic lysis. In adults the disease may be caused by deficiencies of calcium, phosporus or vitamin D in the diet, disturbances in absorption of calcium or vitamin D from the bowel or excessive loss of serum phosphorus from the kidneys. It is essentially a disease of mineralization and there is no interference with organic matrix formation (c.f. osteoporosis in which there is a deficiency of organic matrix formation). As has been explained the two conditions may coexist.

The disease may be associated with bone pain, pathological fractures and even bone deformity. However, the full blown picture is rare in the Western hemisphere. Milder degrees are however, quite common and the condition should be born in mind in elderly patients with fractures particularly if the fractures are repeated or fail to heal.

Radiographs may be difficult to distinguish from those of osteoporotic patients. The bones are more radiolucent than normal, the trabecular pattern may be coarser and focal areas of radiolucency called pseudofractures or Looser zones may be present. Later the cortices become thinner and less opaque and finally bone deformity and pathological fracture may be seen. The serum calcium or the calcium phosphate ratio may be below normal and the serum alkaline phosphatase is raised. In the last resort the condition may be diagnosed by bone biopsy.

TREATMENT OF THE ELDERLY PATIENT WITH A FRACTURE

In general it is desirable to fix fractures in the elderly internally so that they be kept mobile. Before and after surgery, attention should be paid to maintaining the haemaglobin, fluid and electrolyte balance and to prevention of pulmonary and venous complications. Pre-existing medical conditions may require reassessment and energetic treatment.

Devoted nursing care is essential to maintain their well being, their interest in life and to prevent the many complications to which they are prone.

Rehabilitation of the elderly is often a team effort depending on nursing care, patient but firm physiotherapy, home assessment by occupational therapists, arrangement of social services by social workers and finally help and advice from general practitioners and geriatricians.

Regretably, despite all this effort many patients end up permanently institutionalized.

COMMUNICATION WITH PATIENTS

It always pays the clinician to give a little time to discuss with the patient the likely progress of his injury. This will help him or her to accept the time periods involved, the possibility of certain complicating factors which may lead to an alteration in treatment, and finally, to an understanding of what may reasonably be expected to be achieved after treatment of the injury. e.g.:

A patient with a Colles fracture may be warned that the wrist may not be quite the same shape as before despite adequate reduction, and that there may be a prominence on the ulnar side of the wrist in the region of which some pain may be experienced for a month or two after the plaster is removed.

This kind of communication has the patient on your side during treatment and rehabilitation.

If the injury is a bad one tell the patient early but at the same time give encouragement. Remember it is not your fault that he or she sustained the injury but the patient may be looking around for someone to blame. Hence a poor result may be ascribed by him or her to poor treatment. Adequate and timely communication prevents this kind of unnecessary unpleasantness.

Note

The Author expects students to remember constantly that:
1. Multiple injuries are multiple.
2. The most serious complication of any fracture may be an *associated injury* especially if undiagnosed.
3. Always think of possible complications of fractures and of the treatment of fractures. This will keep you out of trouble with examiners, coroners and patients' solicitors.

Part II
The management of individual fractures

Introduction

If the student has studied and understood the preceding pages, he should have acquired most of the information required to diagnose and treat any individual fracture and also to discuss that individual fracture at an examination.

For example any question concerning fracture of the shaft of the tibia could be answered quite adequately from the information in Part I of this book. As an example let us answer the examination question, *'Discuss fractures of the tibial shaft'* from what we already know:

The fracture may be traumatic or pathological, simple or compound, complete or incomplete, comminuted or even a stress fracture.

The four displacements of the fragments can all occur here. History and examination are as described not forgetting to exclude complications and associated injuries. Radiographic examination in two planes. Time necessary for union — about 12 weeks in adults, half as long in children.

Principles of treatment
— First aid.
— Preliminary assessment.
— Treatment of fracture itself.
— Reduction — all the methods are used at times.
— Plaster technique.
— Indications for traction.
— Open reduction of fractures: indications
                                          methods.
— Restoration of function: preventive measures
                                 active use
                                 physiotherapy
                                 return to normal living
                                 and employment.

Brief discussion on principles of treatment if fracture were compound.

Complications:
— associated injuries
— injuries to nerves or vessels
— delayed union
— non-union
— mal-union
— joint stiffness
— pathological ossification (rare)
— reflex sympathetic dystrophy
— fat embolism

What an excellent comprehensive answer this would be!

However, if the question were, 'Discuss fracture of the scaphoid bone' the student would require to know some information particular to this fracture. For example:

Caused by falls on the outstretched hand. Tenderness in the anatomical snuffbox. Not necessarily visible on initial X-rays. Requires immobilization in special plaster cast. Prone to non-union and avascular necrosis. Majority of fractures unite if treated adequately but many do not unite if untreated. Non-union may be surprisingly free from symptoms.

It is therefore the purpose of this book in dealing with individual fractures to emphasize that information which is particular to that fracture. The student will be expected to be able to apply the general principles of fracture treatment himself or herself. There will also be paragraphs concerning technical considerations, mainly for postgraduate students, but what the undergraduate student needs to know is the answer to the question, 'What information is particular to this fracture and distinguishes it from other fractures?'

Fractures of the spine

Practical anatomy

The vertebral bodies and intervertebral discs form a strong mobile column well designed to resist compression forces while allowing flexion, extension, lateral flexions and rotation. However, this column is less well constructed to cope with shearing forces either transverse or rotational. Behind the vertebral bodies connected to them by the pedicles are the paired apophyseal joints. These joints together with longitudinal ligaments, and ligamenta flava, interspinous, supraspinous, intertransverse ligaments etc., supported by postural muscles, are the major protection against shearing forces and control rotational stability. These posterior structures may conveniently be named, 'The posterior ligament complex'.

The spinal cord runs in the canal and ends at the lower end of the first lumbar vertebra. Below this is the cauda equina. For a short distance, from about T10-L2, there are roots and spinal cord running together. It is to be noted that a cord transection at the frequently encountered T12-L1 level will isolate the sacral cord below the transection and hence isolate the bladder centre.

The thoracic spine may be regarded as 'protected' against severe injury by the ribs. Hence the areas most vulnerable to rotational shearing forces are near the junctions between 'protected' spine and 'unprotected' spine. In practice this means the thoracolumbar junction and lower cervical spine.

Classification of spinal injuries (Fig. 5)

1. *Classification by mechanism of injury*.
The forces involved are compression, flexion with compression, flexion with rotation and hyperextension.
a. Compression. This usually produces a simple crush fracture.

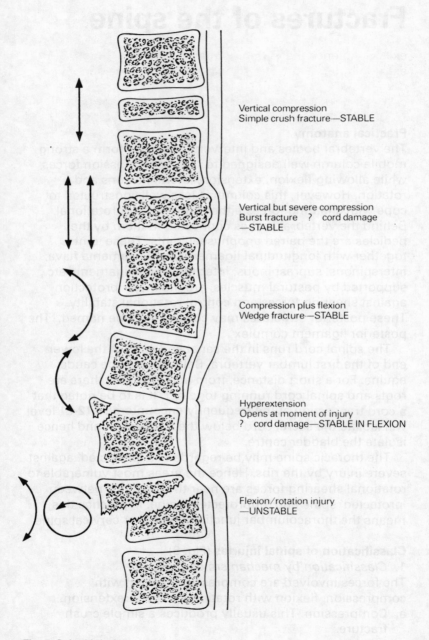

Vertical compression
Simple crush fracture—STABLE

Vertical but severe compression
Burst fracture   ?   cord damage
—STABLE

Compression plus flexion
Wedge fracture—STABLE

Hyperextension
Opens at moment of injury
?   cord damage—STABLE IN FLEXION

Flexion/rotation injury
—UNSTABLE

Fig. 5 Spinal injuries.

b. Flexion/compression. This usually produces a simple
   wedge fracture.
   These fractures are usually stable and innocuous but with
excess violence the vertebrae may be virtually 'burst',
extruding debris posteriorly into the spinal cord and thus
causing cord damage.
c. Flexion/rotation injuries. These produce shearing strains
   that are likely to produce dislocations and fracture
   dislocations. In practice this type of injury is the most
   likely to produce neurological damage.
d. Hyperextension injuries. These are usually caused by a
   fall onto the face with resulting forced hyperextension of
   the neck. The displacement is momentary but injury to
   the spinal cord may be caused.

2. *Classification by stability*
Fractures are either stable or unstable and thus for practical
purposes may be regarded as 'safe', 'potentially unsafe' or
'frankly unsafe'.

3. *Classification by association with neurological damage*
Fractures may occur with or without cord or nerve root
damage. There is a great difference between the treatment
of a fractured spine with cord damage and treatment of a
fracture without cord damage.

**The significance of neurological damage or instability of the
fracture in the management of that fracture**
A stable fracture without neurological damage is easily
managed. Treatment may be as simple as bed rest or
perhaps utilizing a turning bed or even a plaster bed. The
point is that the patient can *feel* and therefore does not
require constant frequent turning to avoid pressure sores.
Such fractures usually heal well with minor after effects such
as aching and weakness of the spine.
   An unstable fracture without cord damage usually
requires more careful attention and some form of
immobilization. The cervical spine can be immobilized in a
plaster cast, by skull traction with later plaster or by 'halo'
splint. The dorsal and lumbar spine can be protected by
careful nursing, turning beds or plaster beds. It is rarely
necessary to perform open reduction and internal fixation.

However, persisting instability may necessitate spinal fusion at a later stage.

A fracture with cord damage is treated with the emphasis on the patient with cord damage rather than on the fracture itself.

Spinal shock
After transection, the segmental and intersegmental activity of the cord below the level of the lesion ceases altogether. This is known as spinal shock. After hours or days reflex activity returns in the isolated cord below the transection.

Let us consider by way of illustration a patient admitted to an Accident Department with a fracture dislocation and cord damage in the lower cervical region.

Immediate problems
1. The patient may have an associated injury, e.g. head injuries are often associated.
2. The patient may require resuscitation as result of other injuries.
3. The patient has transected the spinal cord above the sympathetic outflow. There may thus be a precipitous fall in blood pressure.
4. The patient can only survive if he or she can breathe via the diaphragm (phrenic nerve C3-4). This is less efficient and any other respiratory problem recent or past may cause respiratory failure. Even obesity may prove too much of a load.

    The maintenance of an adequate airway when there is an unstable injury of the neck is in itself a problem.
5. The patient may not be able to control body temperature.

Intermediate problems
1. Following successful resuscitation the next problem is that of care of the patient's skin. The patient cannot feel or move and in addition may not be perfusing the skin adequately. This combination may cause pressure necrosis within a few hours. Therefore, two hourly turning of the patient must be commenced as soon as possible preferably within six hours.
2. The bladder. There is no urgency to deal with the paralysed bladder. However, when overflow

incontinence occurs it is time to catheterize the patient. Immaculate technique is necessary to prevent infection which can doom efforts to produce a well functioning automatic bladder.

Our intention must be to drain and keep clean the bladder until automatic reflex activity returns. The ideal outcome if paralysis persists is for the bladder to remain clear of infection and to empty itself regularly when a certain volume of urine is reached. Paraplegic patients are often able to find trick stimuli to precipitate reflex micturition. This is very important to female patients for whom there is no satisfactory incontinence appliance.

Long term problems
1. Careful positioning and bolstering of limbs prevents contractures developing. Physiotherapy maintains joint movement while recovery is awaited.
2. The bowels may become constipated.
3. The permanently paralysed patient has to be rehabilitated as well as possible. In practice independent wheelchair existence is possible if the patient can lift his buttocks off his wheelchair at regular intervals himself or herself. If this is not possible the patient will require 24 hour a day assistance.

   Paraplegic patients often lead very satisfactory and independent lives and can return to useful employment.
4. The paralysed patient suffers from great social, psychological and sexual problems. These have to be dealt with sympathetically.

Care of the fracture itself
Emphasis has already been made towards the significance of sensation in the management of spinal fractures. In most complete cord injuries, sensation will not be present.

Unstable injuries of the cervical spine
These require immediate immobilization. This can be effected by securing a caliper or pair of tongs to the skull. A variety of these exists but the author prefers those which do not require holes to be drilled into the outer table of the skull. The caliper can be applied using local anaesthetic a few centimetres above and behind the ear.

The traction is used firstly to immobilize the fracture. It is applied in the long axis of the body over a pulley attached to the head of the bed. The patient can then be turned in the axis of this traction. If a dislocation of the spine exists with or without a fracture the traction can be used to 'loosen' the dislocation prior to reducing it by manipulation under anaesthesia i.e. unlocking of locked facets. Usually a weight of up to 10 kilograms will be needed to 'unlock' a cervical dislocation. Once reduction has been achieved the weight is reduced.

The traction is maintained for approximately six weeks after which immobilization can be achieved by a variety of methods. The halo splint is very suitable but as the skin over the neck and shoulders usually has sensation, various collars may be used. Patients without cord damage may have the caliper incorporated into a Minerva type of plaster at this stage or be managed safely with this plaster alone.

Spontaneous interbody fusion will often occur within 3–4 months but persisting instability or pain at the fracture site may require cervical spinal fusion which may be carried out anteriorly or posteriorly.

Unstable injuries to the dorsal and lumbar spine
These injuries rarely require internal fixation. The fracture may be satisfactorily treated in the majority of cases by careful turning in a bed or turning frame. Spontaneous interbody fusion usually occurs. If instability or pain persist, spinal fusion may be occasionally required. However, there are certain indications for exploration, reduction and fixation of the fracture internally.

For example, deterioration in the neurological state some time after the injury may necessitate decompression and fixation. A variety of devices may be used to fix these fractures including spinal plates and Harrington rods with laminar wiring.

In general in the U.K. the practice has been conservative. There is a great pressure on the surgeon to 'do something' for the paralysed patient. Unless there is a specific reason for interference, it is wiser to avoid surgery.

Guides to prognosis
There is no certain reliable way of gauging early what the

chances of recovery of a neurological lesion are. Obviously the degree of displacement of the fracture may give a clue. Reflex activity in certain perineal muscles is sometimes a guide. The most encouraging signs are those of incompleteness of the paralysis, or early return of cord function. The patients with early recovery normally achieve the most recovery.

Fractures of the thorax

Although these injuries are often regarded as 'orthopaedic' the important aspects of management are medical.

Rib fractures usually occur as a result of direct violence. They may be very painful and inhibit deep breathing and coughing, thus leading to pulmonary complications, especially in patients already predisposed to these conditions, e.g. elderly chronic bronchitics.

Treatment consists of providing pain relief initially, encouraging breathing exercises as soon as pain allows and observing the patient for complications.

The complications to be thought of and excluded are: Associated injury, e.g. kidney or spleen with lower rib fractures.

— Pneumothorax
— Haemothorax
— Damage to major air passages with surgical emphysema.
— Pneumonia.

Initially the patients will be radiographed. They should be examined clinically from time to time and it is sound practice to repeat the radiograph after a few days to exclude complications.

Pain relief may be difficult. Intercostal nerve blocks may give temporary relief. Strapping the chest in the damaged area only is a time honoured method and affords comfort to some of the patients. Note that the strapping should never extend all around the thorax. This method is probably inadvisable in those patients who are predisposed to pulmonary infection. Most patients will manage with analgesics but pain and tenderness may persist for some weeks.

Multiple fractures of the rib cage, stove-in chest, flail segment

Where there are multiple injuries to the ribs and or sternum the liklihood of contusion and laceration of the lung, penetration of the pleural cavity and injury to air passages increases. Clinically a watch must be kept for air or blood in the pleura and mediastinal shift. Repeated radiographs and blood gas analysis are invaluable in the early phases.

Flail segment injuries of the chest are of particular importance. When a patient inspires, a negative pressure is created in the chest. The first part of the air inspired will come from the dead space. If part of the chest wall is flail i.e. free to move independently, it will be 'sucked in' on inspiration thus occupying space into which the inspired air should have moved. The inward movement of a flail segment when the rest of the chest is moving outward during inspiration is called paradoxical movement.

These patients may of course have additional damage to lung or pleura and may become rapidly anoxic. It is not within the scope of this book to go into the details of management of serious thoracic injuries. However, three actions in the early stages may be life saving.

1. *Endotracheal intubation*. This reduces the dead space, clears the airway and allows suction.
2. *Drainage of the pleural cavities* (with underwater seal). This manoeuvre gives control of the pleural cavities. Now it may be seen if air is escaping into them or whether haemorrhage is occurring. The lungs remain expanded. Also if IPPR is to be used, this may prevent tension pneumothorax.
3. *Intermittent positive pressure respiration*. Ventilation of the patient will cope with most of the eventualities after a chest injury if combined with intubation and pleural drainage. Even flail segments will be controlled.

The management of serious chest injury may be very difficult. Tracheostomy and even rib cage fixation may have a place in individual cases. Antibiotics and physiotherapy play a part. However the three principles above may be life saving as initial measures.

Fractures of the pelvis

Practical anatomy
The pelvis may be likened to a ring, which includes the innominate bones, the sacrum, the sacro-iliac joints and the symphysis pubis. When fractured, the pelvis tends to break the ring at two places (Fig. 6). If only one fracture is visible, consider the possibility of disruption of a sacro-iliac joint (particularly if the patient complains of backache). The pelvis is very vascular and anteriorly the bladder and urethra are positioned vulnerably.

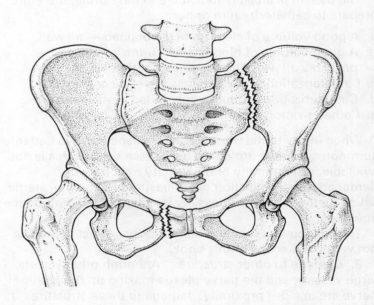

Fig. 6 Typical fracture of pelvis — the 'ring' is broken in two places.

Mechanism of injury

The pelvis is very strong and in most patients a great deal of violence is required to fracture it. Usually this is direct violence of high velocity. As an exception, old ladies with osteoporotic bones may sustain a mild fracture of a single ramus simply by toppling over and crumpling it.

High velocity injuries are often associated with *other injuries* and are often *complicated*.

Early complications and their management

1. *Haemorrhage and shock.* These patients may bleed very severely into soft tissues. Blood loss of 3–4 litres is not uncommon. If the bleeding associated with other injuries is added to this, early severe hypovolaemic shock may be expected. Prepare for urgent replacement of blood loss.

2. *Damage to urinary tract.* Injuries to the urethra and extraperitoneal rupture of the bladder are frequently associated with pelvic fracture. The clinician must establish early that these have not occurred.

The patient is unlikely to be able to pass urine, therefore prepare to catheterize him or her:

a. A good volume of clear urine is obtained — *all well.*
b. A good volume of bloodstained urine is obtained — *probably all well.* Leave catheter and observe.
c. Catheterization proves impossible — *all is not well.*
d. Catheterization produces only blood — *all is not well.*
e. Catheterization produces no urine — *all is not well.*

When injury to the urinary tract is suspected it is better to summon specialist urological assistance early. If this is not available, discontinuity of the urinary tract may be demonstrable by injection of a measured quantity of sterile saline up the urethra or possibly injection of a radio-opaque liquid.

The subsequent management of urinary tract injuries is not within the scope of this book.

3. *Damage to other structures.* Although other viscera, large vessels, and the nerve plexus making up the sciatic nerve are in close proximity, damage to these structures is fortunately rare.

4. *The hip joint.* This is part of the pelvis. Damage to the acetabulum may require treatment.

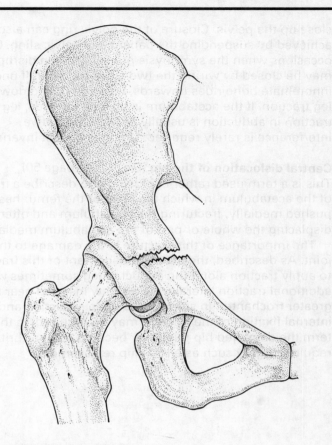

Fig. 7 'Central' dislocation of the hip.

Late complications
These are few. Obstetrical problems rarely arise. A damaged acetabulum may lead to osteoarthritis of the hip.

Management of the fracture itself
You will have noted that this is considerably less important than recognition of and treatment of any complications.

The pelvis tends to open out as a book. Thus placing the patient on a mattress tends to exert a lateral pressure and close up the pelvis. Closure of the pelvic ring can also be achieved by suspending the patient in a pelvic sling. On occasions when the symphysis pubis has been disrupted, it may be closed by wiring the two sides together. If one innominate bone rides upwards, it can be pulled down with leg traction. If the acetabulum is pushed inwards, leg traction in abduction is usually applied. Operative interference is rarely required. Union is almost invariable.

Central dislocation of the hip (Fig. 7: see page 50)
This is a term used rather confusingly to describe a fracture of the acetabulum in which the head of the femur has pushed medially, fracturing the acetabulum and often displacing the whole or part of the acetabulum medially.

   The importance of this fracture is the damage to the hip joint. As described, the usual management of this fracture is to apply traction along the abducted leg sometimes with additional traction laterally via a screw inserted near the greater trochanter. In some cases open reduction and internal fixation of the fracture may be required. In the long term the damaged hip joint may become osteoarthritic and require surgery such as a total hip replacement.

The lower limb

DISLOCATION OF THE HIP

Practical anatomy
The hip is a deep socketed joint and considerable violence is
required to dislocate it. Not surprisingly associated
acetabular fractures are common.

Behind the hip, lies the sciatic nerve in a vulnerable
position.

The capsule at the back of the hip which is inevitably
ruptured in a dislocation backwards, contains important
retinacular vessels supplying the head of the femur.

Mechanism of injury
The majority of dislocations are posterior. They are incurred
by an impact on the knee when the patient is in a sitting
position, e.g. in a car. The impact on the knee may cause
other injuries.

Anterior, inferior and central dislocations also occur but
much less commonly.

Diagnosis
The patient has had a severe injury and may have others.
Patients with dislocated hips often seem shocked until
reduction is achieved.

The affected thigh will be flexed, adducted and internally
rotated as might be expected. A history of injury with pain
and tenderness completes the picture.

Naturally, the diagnosis is confirmed by a radiograph.
Beware!
We have noted that the injury is caused by an impact on the
knee. Hence it is quite common for there to be an associated
injury to the patella or femur. A femoral shaft fracture will
disguise a dislocation of the hip perhaps leading to one of
the great diagnostic disasters of trauma.

It is advisable to insist on a radiograph of the pelvis in all cases with a major injury to the lower limb.

Complications
Early: associated fracture;
         sciatic nerve injury.
Late: avascular necrosis of the femoral head;
         osteoarthrosis of the hip.

Instability in this deep socketed joint is not usually a problem unless there is an associated acetabular or femoral head fracture and therefore recurrence does not occur.

Treatment
The hip must be reduced under general anaesthesia with good muscle relaxation.

It is convenient to anaesthetise the patient on the floor so that the operator may stand over him.

The hip and knee are flexed to a right angle. The deformity is increased and traction is applied in the long axis of the femur. In most cases the hip reduces with a satisfying clunk.

The hip is then rested for six weeks by applying traction to the leg on a Thomas' splint or similar. After this time the patient may be allowed up with crutches non weight bearing on the affected leg for a further six weeks.

If a large bone fragment is displaced from the posterior acetabular margin, open reduction and internal fixation of the fragment may be necessary to ensure stability.

It is advisable to follow these patients as avascular necrosis may appear many months later. Discussion of this possibility may make it easier for the patient to co-operate with the prolonged follow up.

FRACTURES OF THE FEMORAL NECK AND TROCHANTERIC REGION (Fig. 8)

Although there are many differences between these groups of fractures, they share the important common factor of occurring in the same group of patients with the particular problems of that group. They should therefore be considered together.

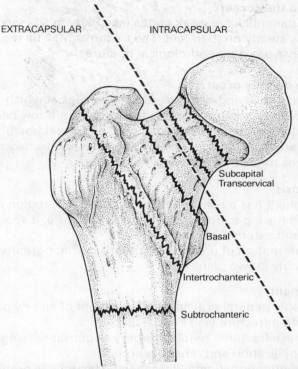

EXTRACAPSULAR   INTRACAPSULAR

Subcapital
Transcervical

Basal

Intertrochanteric

Subtrochanteric

Fig. 8 The sites of fracture of the femoral neck are easy to remember — the descriptions are anatomical. Note that treatment depends on whether the fracture is intra-or extracapsular.

Practical anatomy

The blood supply to the femoral head arrives via three possible routes, in retinacular vessels travelling in the posterior capsule, via medullary vessels in the femoral neck itself and through the ligamentum teres. Of these the first two are much more important and both sources can be damaged when a fracture occurs across the femoral neck.

Note that extracapsular fractures do not damage the blood supply to the femoral head and therefore do not suffer the consequent problems of avascular necrosis of the femoral head and non union.

Who gets them?

These are fractures of the elderly, particularly elderly females.

Why do they occur?

These patients have weak bones (see Part 1 p. 28), and they are less steady on their feet. The fractures may be regarded in a sense as being pathological fractures.

Where do they occur?

The accompanying diagram shows the sites at which femoral neck and trochanteric fractures commonly occur.

Subtrochanteric, intertrochanteric and basal fractures may be regarded as extracapsular. Subcapital and transcervical fractures may be regarded as intracapsular.

Diagnosis

The patient has a history of injury, pain in the region of the hip and the leg adopts a characteristic posture. It appears short and externally rotated.

Confirmation of diagnosis depends on radiographs, preferably in two planes.

Treatment

1. Apply general principles of treatment of elderly patients with a fracture (see Part I p. 30).
2. These fractures require surgery to permit nursing, early mobilization and rehabilitation.
3. In younger patients, (less than 60 years) it is probably advisable to try to conserve the patient's femoral head and pin the fracture.
4. In older patients, pin the fractures which are extracapsular and replace the femoral head of all displaced fractures which are intracapsular. Undisplaced intracapsular fractures may be pinned.

Noteworthy complications

1. Complications of an elderly hospitalised patient undergoing surgery.
2. Avascular necrosis of the femoral head.
3. Non-union of the fracture.
4. Mal-union with varus angulation and shortening.

Technical considerations

A great deal of thought and ingenuity has been devoted to the internal fixation of femoral neck fractures and many methods are available.

Extracapsular fractures require some form of nail and plate fixation. Recently there has been increased enthusiasm for fixed angle nail-plates with compression devices on the nail.

Intracapsular fractures may be pinned in selected cases. Again a nail plate is preferred.

Intracapsular fractures with displacement may require replacement of the femoral head. An Austen-Moore type prosthesis which is punched into the upper end of the femur after reaming may be used. However, a case can be made out for primary total hip replacement in such cases, particularly if the patient is relatively young and fit.

Impacted abduction fractures may be treated conservatively or pinned. It is preferable to pin these with several smaller pins 'spread' into the femoral head. The use of these avoids the danger of displacing the impaction. Serial radiographs should be taken to ensure that disimpaction does not occur. Weight bearing may commence early.

FRACTURE OF THE GREATER TROCHANTER

This injury is of much less importance than the preceding fractures. It may be treated by a period of rest followed by gentle mobilization.

Radiographs may be difficult to interpret and it is probably advisable to repeat the radiographs after a few days in any case where there is doubt as to whether the fracture extends more widely.

FRACTURES OF THE FEMORAL SHAFT

In general terms these are unremarkable fractures and general principles apply:
1. These fractures occur at any age.
2 They are usually the result of severe violence.
3. They may occur at any site and of variable pattern.
4. Complications are as might be expected after study of Part I. However the complication of fat embolism, fortunately rare, is most often seen after this fracture.
5. The fracture is most widely treated by manipulation and traction on a splint. *The student must know what a*

Thomas' splint looks like and how it is used. Internal fixation is also often used in management of this fracture.

6. Union usually occurs in 3–4 months.
7. Rehabilitation with exercise is commenced while on the splint and continued more vigorously when splintage is removed.

Technical considerations

1. *Traction.* (Fig. 9) In children traction may be administered by skin traction and may be balanced or fixed.

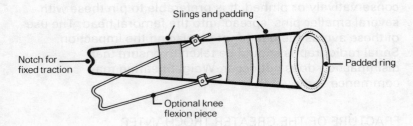

The Thomas splint

Slings and padding

Notch for fixed traction

Padded ring

Optional knee flexion piece

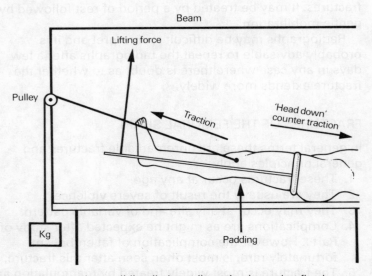

Beam

Lifting force

Pulley

Traction

'Head down' counter traction

Kg

Padding

Fig. 9 The diagram shows sliding (balanced) traction in use but fixed traction — pulling the leg against the ring — can also be used.

Fixed traction is applied from the end of the Thomas' splint against the ring. Balanced traction is usually applied through a skeletal transfixation pin and is taken over the foot of the bed via a pulley as is shown in the accompanying diagram.

In small children under 3 years, Gallows traction may be used from an overhead beam.

2. Once the fracture is 'sticky' external fixation may be used. Traditionally a plaster spica has been the method of choice but more recently widespread use of the method of cast-bracing has been made with considerable benefits to the mobility of the patient. Whichever method is used may permit the complication of late varus angulation and a watch should be kept for this.

3. Internal fixation is possible by a variety of methods. Ideally intramedullary nailing after an accurate reaming of the fragments would be preferred but double plating, single plating and even circumferential banding may be required depending on the shape and size of the fracture.

SUPRACONDYLAR FRACTURE OF THE FEMUR

Practical anatomy
Injuries in region of knee and elbow may damage large vessels.

The gastrocnemii tend to pull backwards the distal fragment (Fig. 10). Therefore immobilization of the fracture with the knee in flexion is desirable.

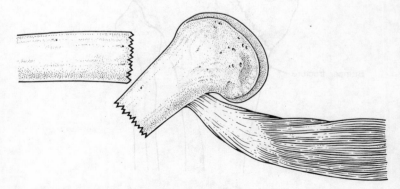

Fig. 10 In supracondylar fractures of the knee, the distal fragment is often tilted backwards by the gastronemii.

Treatment

On the whole these fractures do better with conservative treatment on a Thomas splint with a knee flexion piece added. Internal fixation is possible and may sometimes be indicated.

FRACTURES INVOLVING THE KNEE JOINT (Fig. 11)

Practical anatomy

1. The proximity of the important vessels and nerves behind the knee joint has already been mentioned. *Beware.*

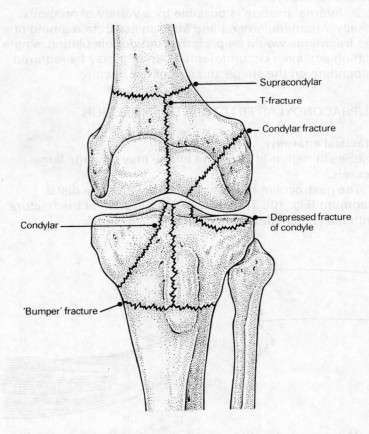

Supracondylar

T-fracture

Condylar fracture

Depressed fracture of condyle

Condylar

'Bumper' fracture

Fig. 11 Fractures around the knee.

2. Weight bearing joints do not tolerate damage or irregularities of articular surfaces well and degenerative disease follows serious injury.

Treatment
1. Painful haemarthrosis may need aspiration for relief of pain.
2. Fractures without displacement or with minor displacement do not require internal fixation. Immobilize appropriately the femur on a Thomas' splint or the tibia in a long leg plaster cast.
3. Minimally displaced fractures of the tibia may alternatively be treated by mobilization while on traction. This ensures early return to full function.
4. Seriously displaced fractures involving articular surfaces need open reduction and internal fixation.

DISLOCATION OF THE KNEE

This is a rare injury. Reduction and immobilization in a plaster cast is adequate. This severe injury is likely to be followed by permanent disability. Beware vascular or peripheral nerve injury. Ligamentous damage is severe. Occasionally immediate surgical repair may be indicated.

FRACTURES OF THE PATELLA

Practical anatomy
1. The patella lies in the centre of the extensor mechanism. It acts as a pulley carrying the mechanism around the knee during flexion. On each side lie the extensor expansions. The patella is thus surrounded by a fibrotendonous 'capsule'.
2. The patella may be fractured by direct violence or by muscle pull or both together.

Treatment
This depends upon whether the extensor mechanism is intact and also upon the degree of comminution of the fracture.

If the extensor mechanism is intact the fractured patella will still retain its 'capsule' and may thus be treated conservatively unless it is severely comminuted. A plaster cylinder is the usual method of splintage.

If the extensor mechanism is ruptured surgical repair with or without patellectomy is essential. In general if the extensor mechanism has to be repaired it is preferabe to retain the patella as patellectomy with extensor mechanism repair is often followed by stiffness.

Severely comminuted fractures with displacement of fragments usually require excision of the patella.

A painful tense haemarthrosis may require aspiration for pain relief.

Other injuries of the extensor mechanism (Fig. 12)
In addition to disruption through the patella and extensor

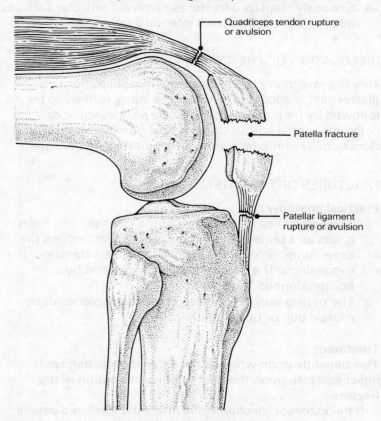

Fig. 12 Injuries to the extensor mechanism of the knee.

expansions the extensor mechanism may be disrupted by avulsion of the quadriceps tendon from the patella, by avulsion of the patellar tendon from the tibial tuberosity or occasionally by rupture of the tendons themselves.

Most cases require surgical repair but some elderly patients may rupture the central part of the quadriceps tendon while retaining the expansion intact. In such cases conservative treatment may be justified.

Lateral dislocation of the patella
This condition may occur singly or as a recurrent problem. It is often associated with some other abnormality such as genu valgum, hypermobile or high patella and shallow intercondylar groove on the femur.

The acute condition is quite dramatic as the patella is visibly displaced. It can be reduced by medial pressure while the knee is gently straightened. The torn medial expansion requires resting in a plaster after which vigorous quadriceps exercises are to be encouraged.

Recurrent dislocation requires surgical treatment, the description of which is not within the scope of this book.

FRACTURES OF THE TIBIAL SHAFT

From the students point of view, these are common but unremarkable fractures. General principles apply as was demonstrated on the opening pages (pp 35–36) of Part II.

Technical considerations
Considerable thought, experiment and effort have been expended over the last decade concerning the best way of managing tibial fractures. It must be said that excellent results are being achieved by completely different methods. A simplified guide to the use of available methods is as follows:

1. Transverse, undisplaced or stable fractures can usually be treated *conservatively in a long leg plaster* (Fig. 13). If manipulation is needed, the author prefers to do this while allowing the leg to hang over the end of the operating table. Gravity now assists maintenance of position of the fragments. Dorsiflexion of the foot must be achieved by traction on the heel and not by forcing up the forefoot,

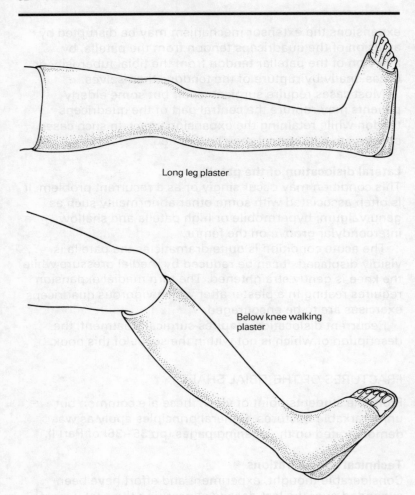

Long leg plaster

Below knee walking plaster

Fig. 13

otherwise the distal tibial fragment will inevitably tilt backwards. While the leg is so held an assistant applies a plaster cast below the knee. The knee is extended and the plaster cast is completed to an above knee plaster, preferably with the knee slightly flexed. The ankle should be at a right angle.

2. *Traction by calcaneal pin* (or lower tibial pin) incorporated in the plaster cast may be used for oblique or

unstable fractures. The pin may be cut and buried in the plaster at three weeks and removed with a change of plaster at six weeks.

3. *Rigid internal fixation by plating with or without compression.* This is a successful method provided rigidity is achieved. Not all fractures allow this, in which case the heavy plates and long incisions used are not advantageous.

4. *Semi-rigid fixation with slightly flexible plates of plastic material.* This has recently been introduced to encourage callus formation at the fracture.

5. *Intramedullary nailing* is an excellent method in practised hands for suitable fractures.

6. *Use of external fixators.* This is a useful method when considerable soft tissue damage is present. Whether its use is justified for simple fractures is doubtful. However, transfixation pins of greater diameter and with tapering seem to remove much of the problem of loosening and pin track infection. If these problems can be overcome with more modern devices, then the method of external fixation may be used more widely for fractures unsuitable for conservative treatment.

ISOLATED FRACTURES OF THE FIBULA

This is an uncommon injury as fibular fracture is more commonly associated with tibial fractures or ankle fractures. However, it can occur as a result of direct violence. In general it is an injury not requiring much more than sufficient support to relieve pain. Often strapping will suffice but a below knee plaster can always be used if pain is severe.

Beware of overlooking the combination of a fibular fracture with diastasis of the ankle.

STRESS FRACTURES OF TIBIA AND FIBULA

Both these bones are the sites of stress fractures. These usually occur in athletes who are training over long distances. The gradual onset of pain and tenderness should make the advising surgeon think of this condition and to search appropriate radiographs for evidence of a hairline crack or for endosteal or exosteal callus.

FRACTURES OF THE ANKLE

Practical anatomy

1. The ankle may be regarded as a ring-like structure composed of bones joined together by ligaments. As a general principle instability results when the ring is broken in two places whether as a result of two fractures or a combination of fractures and ligament damage.

2. The commonest way in which ankles are damaged is by inversion injuries. It is everyone's experience to have turned their ankle at some time or other. What is more difficult to understand is that inversion of the foot is obligatorily linked mechanically with external rotation of the talus. When the tibia is held proximally by postural muscles in such a way that it cannot rotate with the talus, then injuries to the ankle mortice may occur. This is the reason that inversion injuries are classified as 'external rotation injuries'.

3. As a general principle a traction force on a malleolus results in a transverse fracture and a pulsion or rotation/pulsion force results in an oblique or spiral fracture of that malleolus.

A simplified classification of fractures of the ankle

1. *External rotation injuries.*   As explained the talus rotates externally driving against the lateral malleolus.

The mildest injury is a 'sprained' ankle with damage to the anterior part of the lateral ligament. Further rotation may fracture the lateral malleolus of the ankle — the commonest ankle fracture apart from minor avulsion flake fractures. If the force progresses, the medial malleolus may be pulled off leading to a bimalleolar fracture or the medial ligament may be torn. We now have an unstable injury.

Continuation of the rotation may cause a fracture dislocation. If the posterior marginal fragment of the articular surface of the tibia is also fractured we have a trimalleolar fracture dislocation of the ankle and this is the true Pott's fracture (Fig. 14).

2. *Adduction fractures* (Fig. 14). Here the foot is fixed and the talus drives medially knocking off the medial malleolus and pulling off the lateral.

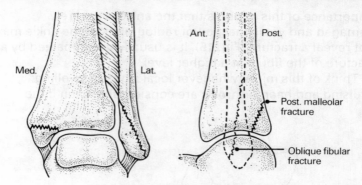

The Potts fracture (External rotation injury)

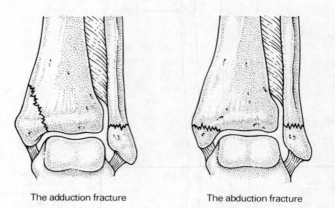

The adduction fracture   The abduction fracture

Fig. 14

3. *Abduction fractures* (Fig. 14). Here the foot is fixed and the talus drives laterally. This fracture bends the rules as both malleoli tend to shear off at joint level.

4. *Vertical compression fracture.* This is really a fracture of the lower end of the tibia involving the articular surface. As a result these fractures are difficult to manage and do badly.

5. *Diastasis of the inferior tibiofibular joint with rupture of the interosseous tibiofibular ligament.* This injury occurs probably as a variation of an external rotation injury. The

importance of this injury is that the ankle is severely
damaged and yet inspection of radiographs of the ankle may
not reveal a fracture (Fig. 15). It is usually accompanied by a
fracture of the fibula at a higher level.

Think of this injury whenever local signs of swelling,
bruising and haemarthrosis are considerable even if the

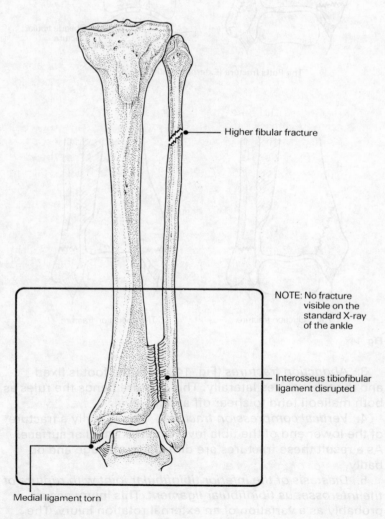

Higher fibular fracture

NOTE: No fracture
visible on the
standard X-ray
of the ankle

Interosseus tibiofibular
ligament disrupted

Medial ligament torn

Fig. 15 The diagnostic pitfall fracture.

radiograph shows no fracture. Examine the radiographs closely for signs of widening of the mortice and palpate the whole of the fibula. If in doubt strain X-rays or examination under anaesthesia may be performed.

This is one of the commonest diagnostic errors from accident and emergency departments. Failure to treat energetically an ankle disrupted by diastasis leads to a very poor result.

Look at the diagram and beware!

Treatment of ankle fractures

It is essential to restore as nearly as possible a normal ankle mortice. Failure to do this results in pain, instability and the early onset of osteoarthrosis.

The first essential is to diagnose the injury. The importance of marked swelling and bruising with tenderness on both sides of the ankle has already been mentioned. Radiographs in two planes will show most fractures and usually show evidence of any diastasis. Routine palpation of the fibula takes little extra time.

Stable ankle fractures may be treated conservatively in a below knee walking plaster usually for about six weeks.

Unstable ankle fractures may be treated conservatively or operatively. If treated conservatively then it is the duty of the attending surgeon to follow these cases carefully with serial radiographs to ensure that displacement does not occur as swelling subsides. Use of an above knee plaster cast may be advisable. Weight bearing must be avoided for four to six weeks.

Many surgeons prefer internal fixation for unstable fractures. This should ensure adequate reconstruction of the ankle and prevent late displacement. Although early weight bearing is still not permitted by internal fixation, mobilization of the ankle while avoiding weight bearing may be started after a few days.

Technical considerations

1. *Plaster of Paris* is still widely used for walking plasters. If allowed to dry for 48 hours it is normally adequate. However weight bearing often causes crumpling of the cast. There is a variety of alternative materials available either to replace plaster or to be used to strengthen

it. This is one of the sites where the additional strength justifies the additional expense involved in their use.

2. *Malleoli* may be internally fixed by *screw fixation or* by *tension band wiring*. If screws are utilized it is preferable to use a malleolar screw designed for the purpose. However, almost any screw may be used provided the malleolar fragment is overdrilled i.e. by a larger drill than the screw so that compression may be achieved.

3. In cases where a *diastasis* is present, the mortice should be closed with *a transverse closing screw*. Care must be taken to tighten this with the ankle dorsiflexed so as to avoid overclosing the mortice.

4. *Posterior malleolar fractures may be left alone* if they are small. Certainly any fragment involving a third of the articular surface or more requires open reduction and fixation.

5. *Fibular fractures* may need *internal fixation* to avoid shortening. This may be by plating, screw fixation, intramedullary rodding or by circumferential wiring.

6. If satisfactory internal fixation is achieved the ankle can be mobilized early, but of course weight bearing is not permitted. Once the ankle is moving well a plaster cast may be applied to protect it in the knowledge that mobilization can be more easily achieved later. Otherwise the ankle is usually immobilized until union is well advanced. Early mobilization of the joint in hospital with the limb elevated is ideal but consideration has to be given to bed availability and the facilities available.

FRACTURES OF THE TALUS

These are rare. The important fact to know about these fractures is that the talus receives it blood supply from distal to proximal. Hence a fracture across the neck of the talus may be followed by the expected problems of non-union and avascular necrosis.

Displaced fractures always require open reduction and internal fixation. Undisplaced fractures may be treated in a below knee plaster. Weight bearing should be avoided until union has occurred and no sign of avascular necrosis is to be seen. However mobilization can be commenced earlier.

FRACTURES OF THE OS CALCIS

The calcaneum is like a chicken's egg, strong when intact but crumples under pressure when cracked.

The calcaneum is usually fractured in a fall from a height. Therefore similar compression injuries may occur elsewhere. Look for and exclude in particular crush fractures of the spine.

The subtalar joint is very complex and it is virtually impossible to achieve full movements of this joint after a fracture of the calcaneum. Hence the aim of treatment is to ensure that the ankle does not become stiff.

The ideal treatment is to rest the patient with the foot elevated and to exercise the ankle from the start. When ankle movements are good and swelling settled, the patient may be allowed up, non weight bearing on crutches. This avoidance of load may be necessary for as long as 10 weeks.

Complications include pain and stiffness at the subtalar joint or spreading of the calcaneum which then abuts on the lateral malleolus.

INJURIES OF THE FOOT

General principles apply here. In most cases conservative management is possible utilizing a plaster cast as for ankle injuries. Dislocations must be reduced and held for six to eight weeks. Irreducible dislocations may require open reduction and fixation.

Fractures of smaller toes require treatment only by the wearing of a strong shoe. Crush injuries of the hallux are common. Sometimes a plaster cast is the most useful treatment and occasionally release of a subungual haematoma may afford great relief of pain.

FRACTURE OF THE BASE OF THE FIFTH METATARSAL

This injury is worth special mention due to its frequency.

Here the common inversion injury is combined with forced plantar flexion at the ankle e.g. misstepping on the edge of a step, stair or pavement edge. The peroneus brevis tendon pulls off the 'styloid' base of the metatarsal bone.

Although the injury appears a minor one, there is often soft tissue damage on the dorsum of the foot and a period of immobilization in a plaster cast is often the surest way to achieve a good result.

STRESS FRACTURES OF THE METATARSAL BONES (MARCH FRACTURE)

Metatarsal bones are another site for stress or fatigue fractures. Typically the shaft or neck of the second or third metatarsal bone is affected.

The patient usually gives a history of prolonged exercise. There is a gradual onset of pain in the forefoot. Local tenderness and swelling on the dorsum of the foot are usually found.

Radiographs often do not show the fracture initially but if repeated will demonstrate the appearance of a haze of callus at the fracture site.

If pain is severe the patient may require a below knee walking plaster (Fig. 13) but mild cases require only a period of rest of the part.

The upper limb

FRACTURE OF THE CLAVICLE

Fractures of the clavicle are unremarkable. They may be caused by direct violence but the majority result from indirect violence, a fall on hand or elbow. They may occur anywhere but usually between the middle and outer third. A smaller number occur at the outer end. Complications are few.

They are treated conservatively by bandaging the shoulders into a 'braced back' position. Traditionally a figure-of-eight bandage is used. Care should be taken to protect the axilla with padding. Union usually occurs in adults within three weeks leaving a visible 'bump' at the fracture site (Fig. 16). Warning the patient about the expected 'bump' ensures good relations.

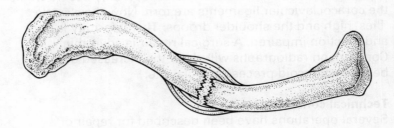

Fig. 16 The fractured clavicle often heals with a 'bump'.

FRACTURES AROUND THE SHOULDER

Practical anatomy

Learn to feel the bony points of your own shoulder. Note that the head of the humerus forms the rounded curve of the shoulder. Note also that it is remarkably anterior. The coracoid process can be felt medial to the humerus and the acromion process above it. The acromio-clavicular joint can just be felt. Behind the shoulder can be felt the spine of the scapula with the infra-spinous and supraspinous fossae.

FRACTURES OF THE SCAPULA

Fractures of the scapula are usually due to direct violence and soft tissue bruising may be extensive. Fractures of the body and neck are usually little displaced because of splintage by attached muscles.

Treatment is by rest, analgesia and mobilization as soon as pain permits. Occasionally a displaced fractured acromion process needs to be excised.

INJURIES TO THE ACROMIOCLAVICULAR JOINT AND CORACOCLAVICULAR LIGAMENTS

The acromioclavicular joint is small and intrinsically unstable. It is thus easily subluxated. This is seen commonly in rugger players who present with a painful 'bump' over the joint. Pain settles in a few weeks with rest and function is restored. A 'bump' however persists.

Complete acromioclavicular dislocation only occurs when the coracoclavicular ligaments are torn. Now the clavicle 'flies' high and the shoulder droops. The deformity is ugly and function impaired. A surgical repair is advisable. Comparison radiographs will show the increased gap between coracoid process and clavicle.

Technical considerations

Several operations have been described for repair of complete acromioclavicular dislocation. The author favours the transfer of coracobrachialis and short head of biceps to the clavicle, a reliable procedure whether the injury is early or late.

DISLOCATIONS OF THE STERNOCLAVICULAR JOINT

This is an uncommon injury. Usually the medial end of the clavicle dislocates forwards. Usually it can be pushed back and in some cases it can be held there by a pad stuck down by strapping. However in many cases it recurs and becomes permanent. Operations have been described for repair of chronic dislocation but the majority of cases do not require this.

Occasionally the dislocation occurs backwards where the clavicle may press on the trachea. This is a rarity but may require open reduction.

DISLOCATION OF THE SHOULDER

Practical anatomy
The majority of dislocations are anterior. Note that here there is a space for the dislocated humeral head to drift medially (subcoracoid) leaving the acromion process as the most lateral part of the shoulder. Much more rarely the dislocation is posterior. Here there is no space to move medially and the humeral head is still lateral but now posterior and palpable in the infraspinous fossa.

Pathology
In younger patients the capsule is strong and the dislocation usually occurs by stripping the labrum glenoidale and attached capsule off the bone leaving a permanent defect into which further dislocations can occur.

In older patients the capsule is burst apart. This will heal after reduction. Recurrent dislocation is thus less common but stiffness may be a problem.

Cause
The majority of injuries are due to indirect violence. Occasionally the shoulder may be dislocated by muscular contraction during convulsive episodes.

Who gets it?
Adults, young or old.

Clinical diagnosis
This is easy. An history and signs of injury plus visible and

palpable evidence of the absence of the humeral head from
where it should be gives the diagnosis. The shoulder has a
square instead of rounded shape (Fig 17).

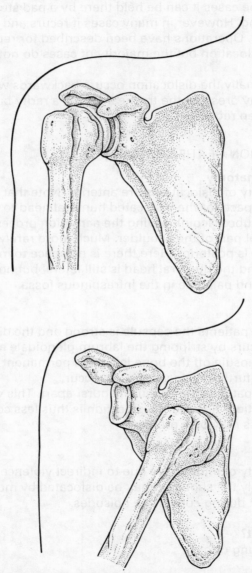

Fig. 17 Note how the shoulder becomes square after an anterior
dislocation.

Radiographs in two planes confirm diagnosis.

Complications

A. *Early*
  1. The axillary nerve may be damaged. Happily the vital structures in the axilla are not commonly damaged.
  2. The shoulder capsule is badly damaged and there may be associated fractures.

B. *Late*
  1. Stiffness. This may occur despite vigorous physiotherapy.
  2. Recurrent dislocation. This indicates permanent damage to the capsule or capsular attachment to the glenoid and may require surgical repair.

Posterior dislocation

This injury is important for two reasons:

First it may be caused by muscle pull during a convulsive episode. Think of this if there is no definite story of injury.

Second it may be difficult to diagnose radiologically. The humeral head does not move medially and therefore on an anteroposterior radiograph it may not appear to be dislocated. Usually a lack of concentricity of the two articular surfaces is apparent. The humeral head has a symmetrical drumstick appearance and the superimposed greater tuberosity may appear as a 'cyst'.

However, clinical diagnosis is easy. The shoulder is not square but the humeral head is missing from its normal anterior position.

Treatment of anterior dislocation of the shoulder

The dislocation is reduced under general anaesthesia or under sedation with intravenous diazepam or similar drug.

With modern anaesthesia muscle relaxation is good and the ancient Hippocratic method of reduction is as good as any. The operator's stockinged foot is placed in the axilla and traction is applied to the semi-abducted arm.

The student may be required to be able to describe the manoeuvre attributed to Kocher. This was useful when speedy anaesthesia was not readily available, but is of less

...he stages of this time honoured
... follows:
... exed to a right angle and traction in the
... erus is applied.
... rotated externally by use of the forearm.
... numerus is adducted across the trunk.
4. The humerus is internally rotated.
   Reduction by any method should be confirmed
   radiologically.
   The limb is rested in a sling for up to two weeks after
which active exercises are encouraged.

INJURY TO THE ROTATOR CUFF

This structure is very elastic, which allows the wide
excursion of movement of the shoulder and is intimately
related to several tendons which run through and help to
stabilise the shoulder. Inflammation of or injury to these
tendons gives rise to various clinical features.

Degeneration of the cuff occurs with increasing age and
sudden strain upon the joint may cause rupture of the
degenerate area — often containing the tendon of a specific
muscle. The most important of these injuries is the
supraspinatus tear.

Minor tears lead to 'supraspinatus tendonitis' and major
tears render the patient incapable of initiating abduction of
the shoulder. Plain radiographs may show calcification but
are usually normal. Contrast medium arthrography may aid
diagnosis.

Major tears in active fit people may require repair.

FRACTURES OF THE SURGICAL NECK OF THE HUMERUS
(Fig. 18)

Cause
Usually direct violence due to fall onto the shoulder.

Who gets it?
Usually middle aged to elderly people, often female.

Diagnosis
History and signs of injury as expected. All fractures of the

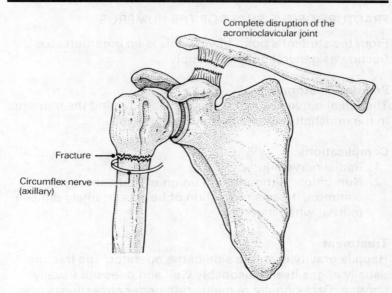

Complete disruption of the acromioclavicular joint

Fracture

Circumflex nerve (axillary)

Fig. 18 1. Fracture of the surgical neck of the humerus.
2. Complete acromio-clavicular dislocation.

upper humerus are accompanied by massive bruising of the upper arm. The seeming absence in some cases of severe pain may be due to impaction of the fracture.

Treatment
Immobilize for 3 weeks with body bandage and collar and cuff sling. Then commence physiotherapy.

In young patients there may be a need for manipulative reduction or even open reduction. Children may sustain a similar injury through the capital epiphysis, a fracture separation.

Complications
1. Rarely the axillary nerve may be damaged.
2. Stiffness is almost inevitable and some or all glenohumeral movement may be lost. Patients compensate well with scapulothoracic movement.

Communication with patient
Warn patient early that it may be difficult to mobilize the shoulder fully.

FRACTURE OF THE SHAFT OF THE HUMERUS

From the student's point of view this is an unremarkable fracture as general principles apply.

Practical anatomy
The radial nerve lies in the spiral groove behind the humerus in the midshaft region and may be damaged.

Complications
1. Radial nerve injury.
2. Non-union. Although non union of this bone is not common, it has a reputation of being extremely difficult to treat when it occurs.

Treatment
Happily gravity is on the side of the operator. The fracture usually aligns itself reasonably well and does not usually shorten. Occasionally manipulation under anaesthesia may be necessary.

Most cases can be treated by seating the patient, supporting the wrist with the elbow flexed and allowing the humerus to hang down by the patient's side. Wool is placed in the axilla and the arm is bandaged to the trunk. Plaster slabs can be stuck on to the bandaging as a shell and moulded to maintain alignment. Alternatively a U-slab may be used, also with the wrist supported in a collar and cuff sling. Some surgeons prefer a hanging cast. Occasionally open reduction and internal fixation may be required using a plate or intramedullary nail.

SUPRACONDYLAR FRACTURE OF THE HUMERUS (Fig. 19)

What makes this fracture so important clinically and so beloved of examiners? It is the importance and number of possible complications.

Supracondylar fractures occur in adults and may require conservative treatment, internal fixation or even skeletal traction. However, it is this fracture in childhood which holds the main interest.

Diagnosis
The child has a fall and presents with pain and a markedly

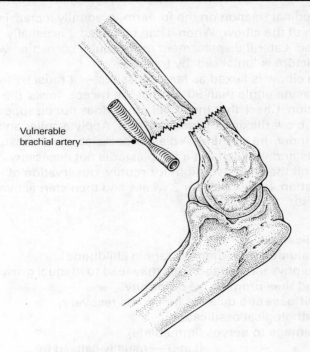

Vulnerable
brachial artery

Fig. 19 Supracondylar fracture of the humerus.

swollen elbow. There is the usual reluctance to use the arm
or to have it moved.

The fracture may be undisplaced, osteochondral and
difficult to see or displaced posteriorly.

X-rays may at times be difficult to interpret, in which case
comparison radiographs of the normal elbow aid diagnosis.

Practical anatomy
Note the position of the triceps muscle. When this taughtens
in flexion it acts as a natural splint to a fracture displacing
posteriorly.

Note the vulnerability of the brachial artery and median
nerve.

Like the shoulder, the elbow has an elastic capsule which
does not tolerate injury well.

Treatment
The fracture is manipulated under general anaesthesia with

longitudinal traction on the forearm, gradually increasing
flexion of the elbow. When it can be flexed it is usually
reduced. Lateral displacement may require correction when
the fracture is 'unlocked' by traction.

The elbow is flexed as far as possible — it must be to a
more acute angle than 90° so that the triceps 'locks' the
reduction. Check that the radial pulse does not disappear
through overflexing the swollen arm. Apply a collar and cuff
sling under the clothing. A plaster backslab may reassure the
parents and yourself but a full plaster is not necessary.

Admit the child overnight for routine observation of
circulation. Immobilize for 3 weeks and then start active
exercises.

Complications
1. Malunion (non union is rare in childhood).
2. Epiphyseal damage. This may lead to inequal growth
   and thus progressive deformity.
3. Stiffness and delayed functional recovery.
4. Pathological ossification.
5. Damage to nerves (Immediate)
                      (Late) — usually caused by
                              progressive deformity.
6. Damage to blood vessels.
7. Osteoarthrosis (late).
8. Reflex sympathetic dystrophy (rare in children).

**Ischaemia of the forearm and hand following supracondylar
fracture in childhood**.
Despite the normally good collateral circulation in the upper
limb, following this injury the forearm and hand can be
ischaemic as a result of:

— Arterial injury with or without thrombosis.
— Arterial spasm.
— Gross intracompartmental swelling.
The clinical signs are:
— Absent pulses.
— Pallor.
— Poor capillary return.
— Excessive pain.
— Inability to permit full passive extension of the fingers.

By the time one sees loss of sensation or paralysis the diagnosis has been too long delayed. In grossly neglected cases gangrene may occur.

Treatment
Preventative: Anticipation and observation prevent this being overlooked.
Active: Remove all bandages, splints etc. Reduce the fracture immediately. Do not overflex a badly swollen arm.

If circulation is not restored in a few minutes summon surgical aid.

The surgeon will decompress the forearm surgically. If this fails to restore circulation a direct exploration of the brachial artery will be required.

Volkmann's ischaemic contracture
This is an entity much loved by examiners.

Following ischaemia of the forearm a block of tissue in the depths of the flexor compartment dies. The skin and superficial muscles survive. The necrotic deep flexors fibrose and contract creating a clawing of all digits.

FRACTURE OF THE LATERAL CONDYLE OF THE HUMERUS

This fracture is important for two reasons:

First it may be underestimated because much of the fragment in young children is cartilaginous. The fracture involves the capitellum, part of the epiphyseal plate and part of the lateral condylar mass. Second the fracture may lead to mal-union or non-union of the fragment. Either eventuality is associated with progressive deformity.

Treatment is along conventional lines.

FRACTURE OF THE OLECRANON

This is a direct impact injury usually treated by internally fixing the olecranon.

Technical considerations
Displaced olecranon fractures are best treated by open reduction and internal fixation with the intention of mobilizing the elbow early. Olecranon screws or tension band wiring may be used.

DISLOCATION OF THE ELBOW

This injury is caused by indirect violence.

It is a serious injury with severe damage to the elbow capsule.

The dislocation is almost always posterior and may be associated with minor fractures of adjacent bones.

The close proximity of major vessels and nerves necessitates careful examination and observation following this injury.

Treatment

Reduction should be performed early as follows:

The patient is placed supine with the arm flexed across the chest. Under general anaesthesia the elbow is flexed gently. Pressure is applied to the olecranon posteriorly until reduction occurs. The arm is rested in a plaster cast with the elbow at a right angle (Fig. 20) for three weeks, after which energetic active exercises must be encouraged. Physiotherapists must be discouraged from stretching the elbow passively.

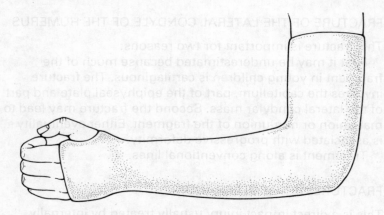

Fig. 20 Full length arm plaster neutral rotation and elbow at 90 degrees.

Complications
1. Vascular injury.
2. Joint stiffness.
3. Myositis ossificans.

FRACTURE OF THE RADIAL HEAD

This is an indirect violence injury. Signs are not impressive but tenderness over the radial head is constant.

Radiographs show the fracture.

Treatment is simple. Immobilize the elbow for two weeks and then commence physiotherapy. If the radial head is severely comminuted excision of the fragments may be the best treatment.

Communication with patient
Warn the patient that full extension will be difficult to achieve after this injury.

FRACTURES OF THE RADIUS AND ULNA

Practical anatomy
The radius and ulna not only connect the hand to the upper arm but they allow the specialized movements of pronation and supination in which the radius rolls around the ulna. Note that the radius is curved for this purpose and note that the two bones are intimately connected by the superior and inferior radio-ulnar joints. The radial head rolls on the capitellum.

Important significance of these facts
1. An injury to the forearm virtually always involves the two bones, or one bone plus one radio-ulnar joint. The only exception is a direct violence injury to the ulna such as might be sustained when lifting the arm to ward off a blow.
   The student must therefore think of injuries to the forearm as double injuries. Hence X-rays of forearm fractures should include the wrist and the elbow.
2. It is important to maintain the correct shape and length of the radius and ulna in order to preserve pronation and supination.

FRACTURES OF THE SHAFTS OF BOTH BONES

These are not remarkable injuries.

In children it is usual to try to treat them conservatively

unless displacement is severe. In adults because of the poor capacity for remodelling it is preferable to err on the side of internally fixing both bones.

Two fractures attract the attention of examiners by virtue of their eponyms, and the fact that they illustrate the double injury concept.

The Galeazzi fracture (Fig. 21)
Fracture in the distal half of the radial diaphysis plus subluxation of the inferior radio-ulnar joint. The fracture is difficult to treat conservatively and internal fixation of radius is usually required.

The Monteggia fracture (Fig. 21)
Here there is a fracture of the shaft of the ulna with dislocation of the radial head. Fixation of the ulna is essential for maintenance of reduction of the dislocated radial head.

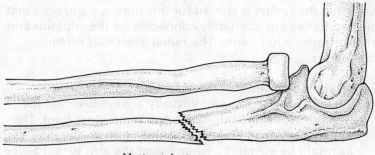

Monteggia fracture

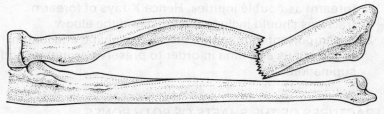

Galeazzi fracture

Fig. 21

Technical considerations

1. *Manipulation of fractures* of the forearm is conveniently done with the elbow flexed and the forearm suspended from the fingers by an assistant. Gravity will assist maintenance of the reduction.

Note that in fractures proximal to the insertion of pronator teres, the proximal fragment will tend to lie in some supination.

2. *Long arm plasters* for fractures of the forearm should be oval in section and thus flattened antero-posteriorly by the operator in the forearm section. 'Round' plasters allow the bones to fall inwards towards each other (Fig. 22).

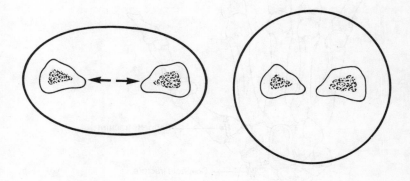

Fig. 22 An oval or flattened plaster cast keeps the radius and ulna apart.

3. A variety of *internal fixation devices* may be used. Intramedullary nailing has its place but most surgeons prefer plating. Whatever plate is used it is always certain that a six hole plate is better than a four hole plate. Semitubular plating has been popular but is often difficult to apply to bones of variable shape and also the plates tend to obscure the view of the bone on subsequent radiographs.

4. *In children* if internal fixation has reluctantly to be performed, little more than a bone suture is required. There is no need for sophisticated plating.

FRACTURES OF THE DISTAL END OF RADIUS

The Colles fracture (Fig. 23)
You must know this one as it is probably the commonest
fracture of all.

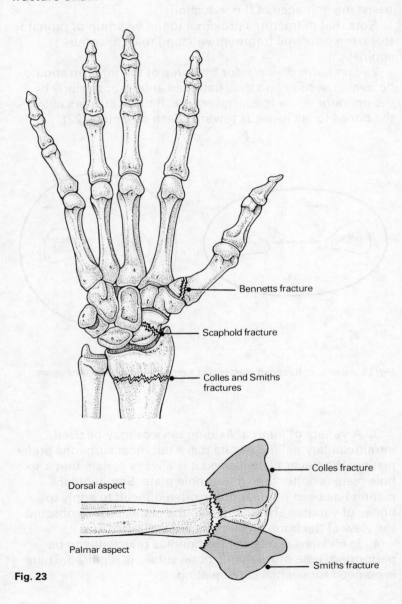

Bennetts fracture

Scaphold fracture

Colles and Smiths
fractures

Dorsal aspect

Colles fracture

Palmar aspect

Smiths fracture

Fig. 23

It follows the rules. The radius fractures in its distal 3 cms with accompanying damage to radio-ulnar joint.

The classic displacement is threefold:

— The distal fragment tilts towards the dorsum.
— The distal fragment shifts towards the dorsum.
— The distal fragment shifs towards the radial side.

These displacements give the classic 'dinner fork' shape (Fig. 24A).

In point of fact the fractures are often comminuted and impacted.

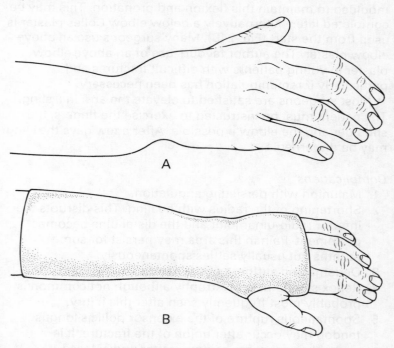

Fig. 24 (A) The typical 'Dinner fork' deformity of Colles fracture associated with radial and dorsal displacement.
(B) Colles plaster.

Who gets this fracture?
It is mainly a fracture of middle aged and elderly patients.

How do they get it?
They fall on the outstretched hand. If you think about it, this is a dorsiflexion-supination injury.

Treatment
Undisplaced or minimally displaced fractures of the distal
end of the radius merely require immobilization in a below
elbow plaster, after which care is the same as for a true
Colles fracture.

A Colles fracture with significant displacement requires
manipulation under general or local anaesthesia. The
fracture is disimpacted by traction and by exaggeration of
the dorsal tilt. The distal fragment is now levered over the
proximal, flexed and pronated. A plaster slab is applied
moulded to maintain this flexion and pronation. This may be
completed later. Alternatively a below elbow Colles plaster is
used from the start (Fig. 24B). Many surgeons use an above
elbow plaster. The author favours use of an above elbow
plaster in young patients with difficult fractures and
particularly if remanipulation has been necessary.

Most surgeons are satisfied to elevate the arm in a sling.
The patient must be instructed to exercise the fingers, the
shoulder and the elbow if possible. After a few days the sling
may be discarded.

Complications
1. Malunion with persisting angulation.
2. Shortening of the radius with healing. This disrupts the
   inferior radio-ulnar joint and the distal ulna becomes
   prominent. Pain in this area may persist for some
   months but usually settles spontaneously.
3. Oedema and stiffness of the hand.
4. Reflex sympathetic dystrophy although not common is
   probably most frequently seen after this injury.
5. Spontaneous rupture of the extensor pollicis longus
   tendon may occur after union of the fracture. It is
   probably even more common after undisplaced
   fractures.
6. Median nerve compression in the distorted carpal tunnel
   may produce the symptoms of carpal tunnel syndrome.
   Mild symptoms are quite frequent but it is unusual for
   surgical decompression to be required.

Communication with patient
Warn the patient that the wrist is unlikely to be exactly the
same shape as the other. Explain about radial shortening

which is not preventable and its effect on the radio-ulnar joint. At the same time encourage the patient by giving an excellent prognosis for function, provided they exercise hard.

The Smiths fracture (Fig. 23)

This is another beloved eponym and therefore important to students. The usage (slightly inaccurately) really covers two fractures. One is the reversed Colles fracture and the other is an anterior marginal fracture of the distal end of the radius with the distal fragment carrying the carpus anteriorly with it.

There is some discussion about the mechanism of this injury. Some cases are due to a fall onto the dorsum of the flexed wrist, such as might occur when a motor cyclist goes over his handlebar. However, the anterior marginal fracture appears to be a flexion-pronation injury.

Treatment

The general principles of treatment are similar to those of a Colles fracture but the reduced fracture is more stable in supination. Hence it is customary to use an above elbow plaster to hold the forearm supinated.

The fracture often occurs in young patients and the outcome is less favourable than in the case of Colles fractures. Because of this some surgeons prefer to treat difficult fractures by open reduction and plating.

FRACTURE SEPARATION OF THE DISTAL RADIAL EPIPHYSIS

This fracture occurs in children and corresponds to the Colles fracture in adults.

The epiphysis slips dorsally usually taking with it a small metaphyseal fragment.

Treatment is the same as for a Colles fracture but immobilization is not required for more than 4 weeks in the majority of cases.

GREENSTICK FRACTURES OF THE DISTAL RADIUS

This is probably the commonest site for 'greenstick'

fractures in childhood. The deformity is similar to a Colles fracture and the distal fragment needs to be held flexed and pronated. It is here that the use of a curved plaster may provide 'three point' correction of the deformity.

Beware the 'springy' greenstick fracture that redeforms within the plaster. In such cases it may often be better to use an above elbow plaster with pronation and 'three point' fixation of the forearm. After 2 weeks the long plaster can be changed to a short one. Union is sound by 4 weeks.

INJURIES TO THE CARPUS

Severe injuries to the carpus occur rarely with various combinations of dislocations and fractures. These require expert attention and often considerable disability results.

DISLOCATION OF THE LUNATE BONE (Fig. 25)

This injury may occur when a fall occurs onto a hand already extended. The lunate is squeezed out to lie anteriorly to its normal position.

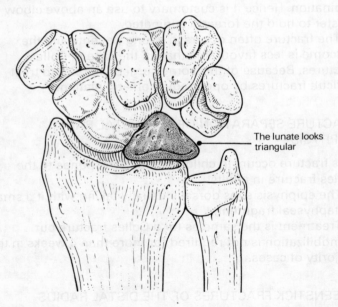

The lunate looks triangular

Fig. 25 Dislocation of the lunate bone.

The diagnosis is usually made radiologically. The lunate on an antero-posterior radiograph normally has a rectangular shape. When dislocated it is distinctly triangular (Fig. 25). Once this is spotted, careful inspection of a lateral film will show its abnormal rotated anterior position.

Treatment is by manipulation under anaesthesia followed by immobilization in a plaster cast. With traction on the hand, direct pressure is applied over the lunate in an attempt to push it back. If this fails open reduction may be required and late cases may be treated by excision of the lunate.

Complications
1. The notable complication is that of avascular necrosis of the lunate because of damage to its blood supply.
2. Osteoarthrosis of the wrist.
3. Median nerve compression.

FRACTURE OF THE SCAPHOID BONE (Fig. 26)

Practical anatomy
The scaphoid is one of those odd bones where the blood supply comes in from distal to proximal. Hence fractures across the body of the scaphoid may render the proximal fragment avascular.

Clinical features
1. The fracture occurs as a result of a fall on the outstretched hand.
2. A painful, swollen wrist with tenderness mainly in the anatomical snuffbox suggests the diagnosis.
3. The initial radiograph may fail to show the fracture. When this diagnosis is suspected, always ask for special 'scaphoid' views of the wrist. Even then the radiograph may be negative.

   Therefore the fracture must be treated on clinical grounds. A repeat X-ray at 2 weeks will probably show the fracture.
4. The fracture is treated in a plaster which includes the metacarpus and the thumb as far as the interphalangeal joint (Fig. 26). Apply the plaster as if the hand were holding a small glass of beer. The plaster is usually retained for six weeks in the first instance.

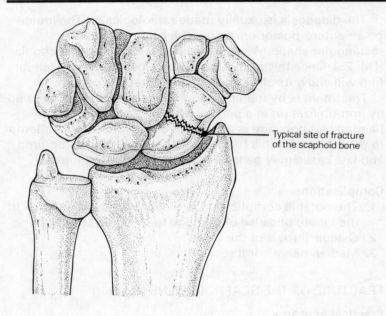

Typical site of fracture
of the scaphoid bone

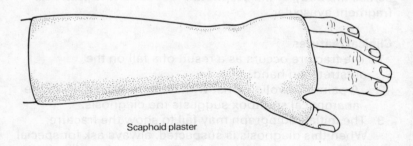

Scaphoid plaster

Fig. 26

Note that fractures of the tuberosity of the scaphoid are much less serious than fractures of the body and usually heal in less than 6 weeks.

Complications
1. Avascular necrosis of the proximal fragment.
2. Delayed union and non-union.

Union may be delayed but by 6 months it should be clear that non-union is present. This may be symptomless in which case it is not essential to interfere. If pain is present some form of bone grafting or fixation of the fracture should be attempted.
3. Osteoarthrosis of the wrist joint.

FRACTURE OF THE TRIQUETRUM

This injury is associated with pain and tenderness at the back of the wrist.

A 'flake' of bone is visible dorsally on the lateral radiograph.

Immobilization in a plaster cast for a few weeks is all that is required.

BENNETTS FRACTURE (see Fig. 23)

This is an eponym which survives and must therefore be learnt.

The fracture is oblique involving the ulnar side of the base of the 1st metacarpal bone. It enters the joint and in many cases is really a fracture-dislocation.

Treatment should be by manipulation and immobilization in a plaster cast similar to a scaphoid plaster. However, it is essential to extend the 1st metacarpal bone by moulding the plaster over felt pads. Note it is not the thumb but the 1st metacarpal that must be extended. If adequate reduction cannot be achieved by conservative means then percutaneous transfixation or open reduction and pinning or screwing of the fracture must be performed.

A transverse fracture of the base of the 1st metacarpal bone can also occur. This is not a Bennetts fracture. It is usually possible to treat this by manipulation and a scaphoid-type plaster.

GENERAL PRINCIPLES IN MANAGEMENT
OF HAND INJURIES

The joints of the hand are vulnerable to oedema and stiffness and indeed oedema leads to stiffness. A united fracture is useless if the hand has lost its mobility. Hence:

1. Prevent oedema by elevation. Serious injuries require admission of the patient with formal elevation of the hand in a roller towel.
2. Encourage early movement. As a rule of thumb, the small joints of the hand should not remain unused for longer than 7–10 days.
3. Immobilize fractures for the minimum time essential.
4. Beware of crush injuries associated with fractures. Stiffness and oedema are a special problem in the crushed hand.
5. The collateral ligaments of the metacarpo-phalangeal joints are stretched in flexion and those of the interphalangeal joints are stretched in extension. Hence the ideal way to immobilize the damaged hand to prevent joint stiffness would be with the fingers straight but flexed at the metacarpo-phalangeal joints. Note that the popular 'boxing glove' bandaging often has the fingers in the reverse state which is not desirable. It is understood that it is not always possible to immobilize the hand in the ideal position but the dangers of a poor position must be avoided if possible.
6. Hand injuries must not be regarded as trivial injuries. Ideally follow up should be at a special clinic where expert advice is possible.
7. Injuries to the small joints of the hand often cause discomfort for many weeks. Mild swelling and pain persist. Reassurance of the patient and encouragement to continue use of the hand will ensure a satisfactory outcome.

FRACTURES OF THE METACARPAL BONES

These fractures may be caused by direct violence or by 'punching' injuries with the fist closed.

Undisplaced fractures may be treated with a light plaster slab and light strapping of the affected digit to its neighbour. Mobilization can be commenced immediately that pain allows.

Displaced fractures may need manipulation, or even internal fixation but this is not common.

Compound fractures of the hand require expert advice initially.

FRACTURE OF THE NECK OF
THE FIFTH METACARPAL BONE

This is a frequent injury, usually caused by a misdirected punch. The distal fragment angulates towards the palm.

Minor displacement requires little treatment. Strapping the little finger to the ring finger and allowing movement is all that is required.

Severe displacement will call for manipulation under anaesthesia. The fracture is then held by splinting the little finger in flexion around a small roll of gauze. A malleable splint may also be used. Note that this fixation may well lead to stiffness and it should not be prolonged.

The fracture tends to heal with slight loss of prominence of the relevant knuckle and a bump on the dorsum of the hand. Function, however, is excellent even with slight persisting deformity.

FRACTURES OF THE PHALANGES

Practical anatomy

The proximal phalanx is surrounded by delicate and complex flexor tendons and extensor tendons. The lumbrical and interosseus muscles are inserted into the extensor hood on the dorsum. Damage to these or interference with their movement will cause loss of function.

Rotational deformities of the fingers may pass unnoticed when the finger is extended. However, when flexion occurs a rotational deformity will cause the finger to cross the palm and interfere with the flexion of its neighbour.

Treatment

On the whole, undisplaced fractures may be satisfactorily treated by strapping of the injured finger to its neighbour.

Displaced fractures may require manipulation and immobilization on a splint (padded aluminium splints are usually favoured). Compound fractures and displaced fractures of the proximal phalanx require special attention and often require internal fixation.

Fractures of the terminal tuft of the distal phalanx should be ignored and any soft tissue injury treated on its merit.

Fractures involving the interphalangeal joints themselves may need special attention and temporary internal fixation may be required.

DISLOCATIONS OF THE METACARPOPHALANGEAL AND INTERPHALANGEAL JOINTS OF THE HAND

These are nearly all due to hyperextension injuries. The distal bone dislocates posteriorly.

Reduction can usually be achieved by gentle traction and pressure over the head of the proximal bone anteriorly. After reduction has been confirmed by X-ray, strapping to the adjacent finger and immediate mobilization is all that is required.

Occasionally the proximal bone may 'button hole' the capsule and be irreducible. Open reduction is required.

MALLET FINGER INJURY

This injury is really an avulsion of the insertion of the extensor tendon into the base of the distal phalanx. It may involve a flake fracture or may be through the tendinous insertion. In general it is easier to manage the cases with an avulsed flake of bone.

The injury is caused by stubbing the finger when it is actively extended. Forced passive flexion causes the avulsion.

The finger adopts a position in which the distal phalanx is flexed. Some evidence of injury to the dorsum of the distal interphalangeal joint is often visible.

Treatment is by immobilization of the distal two phalanges of the finger in a 'mallet finger' splint. Immobilization may need to be continued for six weeks. However, even if healing does not occur, disability is minimal.

ULNAR COLLATERAL LIGAMENT RUPTURE OF THE FIRST METACARPOPHALANGEAL JOINT

This injury is mentioned because it is often overlooked and it is a disabling injury because pinch grip is impaired.

Thus if a patient presents with a painful swollen joint at

the base of the thumb after injury it is advisable to test the integrity of this ligament. Examine it in extension of the joint and compare it with the normal side.

Early complete rupture is best repaired as soon as possible. Chronic or neglected cases are often seriously inconvenienced with persisting pain and weakness. Various methods of repair are possible but in severe cases arthrodesis of the joint gives the surest result.

Ligament injuries

GENERAL PRINCIPLES FOR TREATING LIGAMENT INJURIES

1. *Partial tears* of a ligament may be expected to heal with 3–6 weeks adequate immobilization.

2. *Complete tears* may be associated with permanent instability of a joint. It is better therefore to make the diagnosis early. Often an injured joint (for example a tear of the medial ligament of the knee) may be so painful that the patient will not tolerate attempts to examine and to take strain radiographs of the joint. In such cases it is better to examine the joint under anaesthesia than to miss instability.

3. *A complete tear with demonstrable instability* requires early surgical repair. In practice we are thinking mainly of ankle and knee.

4. *Chronic injuries* (i.e. usually improperly diagnosed initially) may require sophisticated surgical repairs beyond the scope of this discussion.

5. Try to exclude *associated injuries* such as meniscus tears in the knee or extensive capsular damage.

LIGAMENT INJURIES TO THE KNEE JOINT

Soft tissue injuries to the knee are often multiple and early diagnosis is difficult. Combination injuries occur such as the classic medial ligament, medial meniscus and anterior cruciate ligament injury. The ligaments are intimately related to the joint capsule and capsular injuries are commonly associated. Certain clinical entities are usually described.

Tear of the medial ligament
Here an abduction strain on the tibia ruptures the medial ligament (often in association with other injuries as described).

The medial ligament is a long structure and may rupture at its upper end, at the joint line or below the joint line.

Clinically the patient presents with a painful swollen knee with tenderness maximal over the site of the tear. Pain may not allow demonstrable opening of the knee when a valgus strain is applied. However, if this injury is suspected it is worth performing an examination under anaesthesia. In partial tears a painful tense effusion may require aspiration.

Complete rupture should be repaired early followed by immobilization for six weeks in a plaster cylinder. Partial tears may be treated conservatively for three weeks in a similar plaster. It is advisable to follow immobilization with a period of physiotherapy and to remember the possibility that other structures may have been damaged giving rise to further symptoms.

Tear of the lateral ligament
It is doubtful whether isolated injuries of this ligament occur. Management of instability on the lateral side of the knee is similar to that on the medial. Instability is rare because the biceps femoris tendon which is inserted into the head of the fibula helps to stabilize the lateral side of the knee.

Tear of the cruciate ligament
The anterior cruciate ligament is usually torn by hyperextension or forward movement of the tibia on the femur in the flexed knee. The posterior cruciate ligament is torn by a force drawing the tibia backwards on the femur when the knee is in flexion.

These lesions are often associated with a feeling of giving way and instability in the knee. Examination with the patient supine, the knee flexed and the muscles relaxed will show that the tibia can be pulled forward or displaced backwards on the femur more than can be shown on the normal side. The clinical presentation is often influenced by associated injuries.

An 'isolated' cruciate ligament tear does not usually require specific treatment. Repairs are not reliably successful. It is preferable to concentrate on building up the patients' quadriceps muscles by physiotherapy. Most patients learn to live happily with this damaged knee.

The concept of rotatory instability
It used to be said that giving way and locking of the knee

were either due to loose bodies in the knee or tears of the menisci. More recently it has been shown that the combination of ligament tears plus capsular tearing may allow rotatory instability. This implies that the tibia subluxates forward on the femur momentarily when the tibia is rotated on the femur. The patient experiences a sensation of giving way whenever he twists on the knee in a particular direction.

Examination of the knee may show evidence of old injury or cruciate laxity but it requires considerable experience to be able to perform the clinical tests for rotatory instability.

The student is asked to remember that the condition exists and by thinking of it to avoid indescriminate removal of menisci. The patient with rotatory instability will certainly not be improved by meniscectomy.

LIGAMENT INJURIES TO THE ANKLE JOINT

Sprained ankle
As has been previously described, the anterior fibres of the lateral ligament of the ankle may be torn during an inversion injury to the ankle.

Usually pain, swelling and tenderness are well localized below and in front of the lateral malleolus.

The condition may be treated in a variety of ways. Simple bandaging and strapping help most cases. Sportsmen are often treated energetically with physical medicine techniques. More severe cases may benefit from the use of eversion strapping or even a short spell in a walking plaster.

Chronic sprain of the ankle
This clinical entity refers to a condition where, following an ankle injury, the patient experiences repeated episodes of going over on the ankle (i.e. instability) associated with pain and swelling often lasting a few days.

Some of these cases can be shown to have frank lateral ligament insufficiency but the majority do not have such dramatic pathology.

Investigation includes plain radiographs of the ankle and the use of stress inversion films. The latter technique involves the taking of antero-posterior radiographs of both ankles when they are held in forced inversion. The abnormal side can be compared with the normal and if there is gross 'opening' of the ankle on the lateral side, then it is reasonable to assume that the lateral ligament is incompetent.

The average case can usually be treated with a course of physiotherapy including inversion-eversion exercises.

Complete rupture of the lateral ligament

This is an uncommon injury and is often not diagnosed until it is in the chronic stage.

An inversion sprain followed by very severe pain, bruising and swelling may give a clue to the diagnosis. Plain radiographs are usually normal but sometimes an avulsion flake fracture may be seen. Stress films (which may require an anaesthetic) will show 'opening' of the ankle with a talar tilt.

Most cases can be satisfactorily treated in a below knee walking plaster for six weeks. Some surgeons are enthusiastic about early surgical repair. Chronic cases demonstrating instability will require a surgical reconstruction of the lateral ligament.

Meniscus tears

GENERAL PRINCIPLES OF DIAGNOSIS AND TREATMENT
OF MENISCUS TEARS IN THE KNEE JOINT

1. The patient gives a story of injury usually with an element of 'twisting of the knee'.
2. The pain may or may not be well localized but if it is the diagnosis is made easier.
3. The patient is initially disabled, i.e. he does not continue playing football.
4. The knee is swollen and painful often with tenderness over the torn cartilage.
5. The knee will settle down gradually if rested or immobilized and the patient may think all is well.
6. The second or chronic phase of the symptom pattern now appears. The classic presentation is of recurrent episodes of pain and swelling with giving way or locking of the knee.
7. Medial meniscus tears are 5–6 times as common as lateral meniscus tears and are easier to diagnose as they more often give a 'classic' story.
8. The plain radiograph is likely to be normal.
9. Doubtful cases may be investigated radiographically by contrast medium arthrography or the knee may be directly inspected through an arthroscope.
10. A severely torn meniscus does not heal and therefore meniscectomy is usually necessary. It is probable that minor injuries to the menisci often remain undiagnosed.

Pathology of meniscus tears (Fig. 27)
Tears of the semilunar cartilage are usually inflicted by twisting forces when the knee is partially flexed bearing weight and often with a valgus or varus strain in addition.
  There is a line roughly centrally down the long axis of a meniscus where tearing predominates. Complete tearing

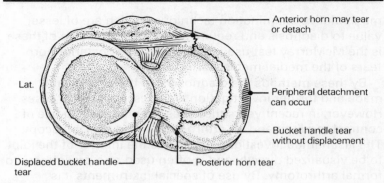

Anterior horn may tear
or detach

Lat.

Peripheral detachment
can occur

Bucket handle tear
without displacement

Displaced bucket handle
tear

Posterior horn tear

Fig. 27 Injuries to the menisci.

virtually divides the meniscus into two. The inner section
can then flip over (like the action of a bucket handle),
obstruct the joint and give rise to the features of a 'bucket
handle' tear. Less severe injuries cause tags either anteriorly
or posteriorly and frequently horizontal cleavage lesions
may be found.

Clinical features

The patient gives a story of injury. Often the injury is well
described but sometimes it is vague. Examination in the
acute phase reveals merely a painful swollen knee with
tenderness over the joint line on the damaged side.
Sometimes the knee is locked which makes the diagnosis
almost certain. Care must be taken to distinguish this injury
from a ligament tear which may require urgent surgery. The
radiographs are negative.

Usually the knee is treated with some form of pressure
bandaging and gradually settles down. When the patient
becomes more active again the classical symptoms of
episodes of pain, swelling, giving way and locking appear.

Examination in the chronic phase will show definite
physical signs. The quadriceps muscles are usually wasted,
there is likely to be an effusion in the knee, there is
tenderness over the affected meniscus in the joint line. The
examiner may be fortunate enough to witness the knee
locked but a much more frequent finding is the loss of the
last few degrees of extension and hyperextension. This is
often described as a 'springy block' to extension, which is a
good description of the physical finding. There are various

manipulative examination techniques which are of lesser value to diagnosis and require some expertise. One of these is the McMurray test used for diagnosis of posterior horn tears of the medial meniscus.

By these methods the diagnosis can be fairly reliably made and further investigation is not essential in all cases. However, in recent years there has been increasing use of contrast medium and air arthrography and of arthroscopy. The last named investigation permits the interior of the joint to be visualized directly and is often used as a preliminary to formal arthrotomy. By use of special instruments it is possible to perform surgical procedures in the knee joint under arthroscopic vision without having to open the joint formally.

Treatment of the acutely locked knee consists of manipulating it under general anaesthesia. This should not be regarded as anything more than a temporary measure which allows reasonable comfort until the patient can be investigated and treated as above.

Part III
Orthopaedics

The orthopaedic consultation

HISTORY TAKING

At least half the common orthopaedic conditions can be diagnosed on the history alone. In brief the history should establish:
1. Exactly what is the patient complaining of. The description of a vague symptom can sometimes be difficult even for articulate individuals. The patient may not be using the same terminology, e.g. by 'pain in the hip' the patient may be indicating buttock pain or groin pain or pain in the region of the greater trochanter or iliac crest.
2. If pain is the complaint ask the usual secondary questions:
   ? Site
   ? Duration
   ? Nature of pain
   ? Continuous or intermittent
   ? Aggravating or relieving factors
   ? Relation to posture and activity
   ? Radiation or referral of pain.
3. Always ask if trauma has occurred.
4. Always ask if any other joints are involved.
5. If swellings are present, always ask if there are any others.
6. Symptoms referring to stiffness, instability or loss of function of a joint will often be best elicited by reference to function, e.g. stiffness of the hip is often best indicated by asking whether the patient can put his shoes on easily.
7. It is important to know the demands of the patients' job, family commitment, sports, recreations etc.
8. Always ask about past treatment. It is not uncommon to find that the patient has already had a consultation elsewhere with radiographs, investigations and a course of treatment.

9. Past medical history is of course important. Think
    particularly of the five carcinomas which metastasize to
    bone: breast, bronchus, thyroid, prostate and kidney.
10. Ask briefly after the patients' general state of health.
11. Remember that symptoms in limbs may have a
    neurological or vascular cause.

EXAMINATION

Examination of superficial joints such as the wrist, elbow
or ankle is simple and speedy and requires only a systematic
routine. However, examination of larger and deeper joints,
e.g. hips and spine is more difficult. The joints cannot be
directly inspected or palpated and much information has to
be inferred. For these joints a special technique is required.

It is more logical in musculoskeletal disease to examine
the affected part first. The patient finds it a little odd if you
spend time examining everything else except the affected
part. A general examination can be made afterwards.

EXAMINATION OF 'SUPERFICIAL' JOINTS

Inspection (compare with other side)
1. Evidence of previous disease — scars
    — sinuses
2. Signs of inflammation — redness
    — swelling
3. Deformity of bones and position of joints

4. Generalized or localized swelling or masses
5. Effusion into joints
6. Muscle wasting

Palpation
1. Signs of inflammation — heat
    — swelling
    — tenderness
2. A lump — situation, size, shape, consistency, surface,
    edge, relations, attachments
3. Synovial thickening or joint effusion

4. Bony landmarks and any deformity
5. Muscle tone and bulk

Measurement
1. — True and apparent length
2. — Girth
3. — Deformity

Movements — active and passive
Usually extension is regarded as 0 degrees and flexion measured in degrees from this. In certain cases it is more convenient to measure other points, e.g.
1. Buttock-to-heel distance to measure full flexion of knee.
2. Fingertip reach down leg to indicate range of flexion of lumbar spine.

Experience will teach that some joints are more usefully assessed by active movements and some by passive, e.g. a fat elderly lady with a painful hip will not be able to demonstrate anything like the range of movements of the hip actively compared with the much more accurate range of movement elicitable by the examiner.

Assessment of ligaments and stability

Assessment of gait and function

Assessment of power and sensation

Assessment of peripheral circulation

Radiography

1. General density or rarefaction
2. Local density or rarefaction
3. Integrity of cortex
4. Joint surfaces
5. Joint spaces
6. Soft tissue

Other special investigations

Radiography and other imaging
 Tomography
 Bone scan (radioisotope scanning)
 Myelography/radiculography
 Arthrography
 Angiography

Computerized axial tomography (CAT scan)
Magnetic resonance imaging (MRI)

Electrodiagnostic
Electromyography
Nerve conduction studies

Blood tests
Common ones are:
Full blood count and ESR
Serum calcium and phosphate levels
Serum alkaline and acid phosphatase
Serum protein electrophoresis
Serum uric acid
Rheumatoid factor
Antinuclear antibodies

Arthroscopy
Direct inspection of the interior of a joint may be made by use of an arthroscope under local or general anaesthesia.
Synovial biopsy — histology

EXAMINATION OF THE HIP — SPECIAL FEATURES

History

Think of back-buttock-leg pain as a symptom complex and try by the end of the history to know which structure is causing the pain.

If the hip joint appears to be the culprit try to elicit the following information:
1. Pain — details of pain as before. Typical hip joint pain is in the groin and referred to thigh and knee.
2. Stiffness — Q. Can you put on your stockings, get into the bath, cut your toenails, get your legs apart etc.?
3. Instability — Q. Do you limp?
4. Deformity — Q. Are your legs the same length?
5. Function — Q. Can you walk, run, negotiate stairs etc.?
    Try to elicit how much the pain is bothering the patient, e.g. does it disturb their sleep?
    Ask about the state of the back, the other hip and the knees.
    Ask about general health, medication and fitness for surgery.

Examination

1. The first physical signs you will notice are the gait:
   a. Short leg gait: The patient bobs up and down. The good knee may be flexed slightly.
   b. Painful leg gait (Antalgic): Everyone knows this gait. If you stand on a tack or twist your ankle you may walk like this for a while.
   c. Stiff hip gait: This is difficult to spot if the patient is clothed. The stiff leg is slid forward by unwinding the lumbar lordosis and flexing the lumbar spine. The pace is then made by extending the lumbar spine.
   d. Instability gait: As the patient takes a step with the diseased hip the centre of gravity of the trunk is thrown over that hip. If bilateral, this gait becomes a waddle (Trendelenburg gait).
2. How does the patient sit down?
   Patients with a stiff hip tend to slouch in the chair slightly and keep the diseased hip close to the front of the chair. They do not sit bolt upright with the knees and hips flexed at a right angle. The diseased leg is either extended fully (males usually) or acutely flexed at the knee (females usually).
3. Next — ask the patient to undress to underpants in males and 'bra' and pants in females. You cannot examine a back or a hip through gaps in outer garments.
4. Ask the patient to stand in front of you with back towards you. Inspect the lumbar spine briefly. Ask the patient to lift each leg off the ground in turn. In normal patients the pelvis lifts on the side of the lifted leg. To achieve this the patient must have a good hip on the side on which he or she is standing. If the pelvis sags instead of lifting, this is the Trendelenburg sign and corresponds to the Trendelenburg gait (Fig. 28).
   Think of 'power', 'fulcrum' and 'levers' and you have a summary of why the Trendelenburg sign may occur:
   Power — weak gluteal muscles
   Fulcrum — diseased hip
   Levers — deformity of upper femur
5. Ask the patient to get up onto the couch and watch how he or she does it. Is it painful? Is it awkward?
6. Inspect the hip, thigh and knee as usual.
7. Palpate the hip, thigh and knees as usual.

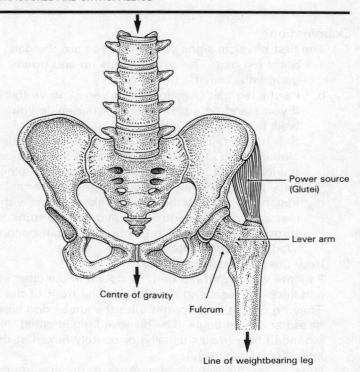

Power source
(Glutei)

Lever arm

Centre of gravity

Fulcrum

Line of weightbearing leg

Fig. 28 Diagram to illustrate the forces involved in standing on one leg and thus the potential causes of an unstable gait and positive Trendelenburg sign.

8. Deformity — the common deformities of hip disease are flexion, adduction and external rotation.
    External rotation is immediately apparent.
    Adduction may be concealed by a pelvic tilt. This can be shown by measuring true and apparent leg length (Fig. 29). Fixed flexion deformities are concealed by lordosis of the lumbar spine. To demonstrate the deformity thus it is necessary to unwind the lumbar lordosis by forcing the good leg up until the pelvis rolls and the diseased leg then flexes up to its deformed position. This is Thomas' Hip Flexion Test. However, if the patient is very fat or the hip very painful he or she will resist your examination and a false assessment will result. The author suggests a modification of Thomas' test in which both legs are flexed up fully, the good leg held and the patient asked

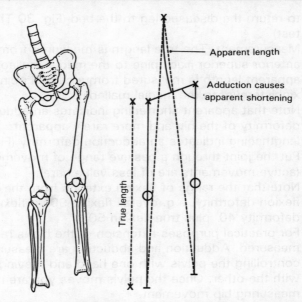

Apparent length

Adduction causes apparent shortening

True length

Fig. 29 Note how fixed pelvic obliquity or fixed adduction deformity can cause apparent shortening of the lower limb.

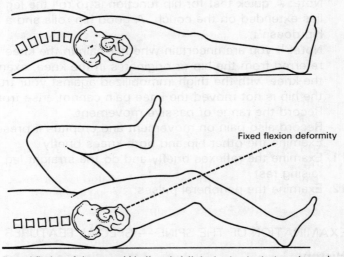

Fixed flexion deformity

Forced flexion of the normal hip "unwinds" the lumbar lordosis and reveals concealed fixed flexion

Thomas' test for fixed flexion at the hip.

Lordosis of the lumbar spine conceals fixed flexion of the hip

Fig. 30

to return the diseased leg to the bed (Fig. 30 Thomas' test).

9. Measurement. The true length is measured from the anterior superior iliac spine to the medial malleolus. The apparent length is measured from a central point, e.g. xiphisternum to the medial malleolus.

    Note that apparent shortening indicates an adduction deformity of the hip and more rarely apparent lengthening indicates an abduction deformity (Fig. 29).

10. Put the joint through a passive range of movement (active movements are of less value here).

    Note that the range of flexion extends from the point of flexion deformity, e.g. overall flexion 90° = flexion deformity 40° plus true flexion 50°.

    For practical purposes extension of the hip is rarely measured. Adduction and abduction are measured by controlling the pelvis with one hand and moving the leg with the other. Once the pelvis moves you are no longer measuring hip movement.

    Internal rotation and external rotation are measured in flexion and extension.

    Note: A quick test for hip function is to roll the leg as it lies extended on the couch. A good hip rolls and a bad hip doesn't.

    Note: If you are uncertain whether pain in the knee is referred from the hip or originates in the knee, examine the knee with the thigh immobilized against your trunk. If the hip is not moved the knee pain cannot arise from it! Record the range of passive movement.

    Record also pain on movement and crepitus if present. Examine the other hip and both knees briefly.

11. Examine the reflexes briefly and do the straight leg raising test.

12. Examine the peripheral pulses.

EXAMINATION OF THE SPINE — SPECIAL FEATURES

History

In addition to general history taking, the clinician must pay special attention to previous backache or trauma. A history of stiffness or other joint involvement may indicate a more generalized joint involvement, e.g. ankylosing spondylitis.

Particular attention must be paid to neurological symptoms. Pain may be referred to a limb, or radiate down a limb due to nerve root irritation. It is not always possible to distinguish between the two but in general true radicular pain is better described by the patient. Ask also about bladder function — any disturbance of this heralds a potential disaster.

General history should not only consider the five carcinomata metastasizing to bone but also visceral disease, gynaecological disease and vascular disease.

Examination
1. Note how the patient walks in and sits down. Patients with severe backache have cautious movements.
2. Ask the patient to undress to underpants in males and 'bra' and pants in females.
3. Ask the patient to stand in front of you with his or her back towards you. Inspect the back as usual with the patient erect and then look along the back with the patient flexed. Asymmetry or a hump on one side indicates a rotational deformity, probably a structural scoliosis.
4. Is the patient balanced? i.e. is the base of the neck over the sacrum? If not, can you see a visible tilt to one side? This may be accompanied by visible muscle spasm and we call this a 'total' or 'sciatic' scoliosis (Fig. 37).

Deformities
The normal spine has a gradual dorsal kyphosis (a curvature convex posteriorly) and a lumbar lordosis (a curvature convex anteriorly). There is a great variation between individuals, sexes and races.

An increase in dorsal kyphosis, if gradual, rarely indicates serious pathology but an angular kyphosis always does. An angular kyphosis indicates bone collapse anteriorly.

Note that flattening of the lumbar spine or loss of lordosis is akin to a kyphosis higher up.

Movements
Active movements are observed and if necessary measured. In ordinary clinical practice it is not necessary to

measure flexion very accurately, e.g. by measurement between spinous processes. A note of the distance down the legs which can be reached by the patient will suffice. Note that there is a considerable individual variation.

The patient is asked to flex, to extend and to flex laterally to left and right. Rotations to left and right largely reflect the health of the dorsal spine. The cervical spine flexes, extends, laterally flexes and rotates freely.

Think of neck–shoulder–arm pain as a clinical entity and always examine the shoulders briefly with the neck.

Pain on flexion of the lumbar spine is more likely to be discogenic and pain on extension to be arthrogenic, i.e. posterior intervertebral joint disease.

Observation of extension and hyperextension is important. Flexion and extension are compounded of rolling and unrolling the lumbar spine and of flexion and extension at the hip. The two movements should occur harmoniously. Abnormalities of extension usually indicate posterior intervertebral joint disease and manifest as:
1. Total instability: the patient has to climb up his legs with his hands to extend.
2. Partial instability: the patient demonstrates a sudden lateral deviation during extension — an instability 'wriggle' or a 'jacknife' movement.
3. Inability to hyperextend.
4. Pain on extension or hyperextension.

Examination prone supine
Ask the patient to get up on the couch and observe how he or she does it. A patient who 'leaps up' onto the couch probably does not have serious pain or pathology. (Similarly note how the patient rolls over.)

Examine the patient in the prone position. Palpate the vertebral spines, the interspinous ligaments and the sacro-iliac joints. Elicit and record any tenderness.

It is convenient while you have the patient prone to test sensation in the saddle area and around the anus. Buttock muscle tone may be tested by asking the patient to squeeze the buttocks together and balotting the buttock muscles with fingertips. Buttock muscle wasting can be well demonstrated by this method.

Ask the patient to roll over (noting how he or she does

it). Flex the hips briefly and roll the legs in extension to ensure good hip function.

Perform the straight leg raising test (having first ensured that the hips are normal). Lift the leg straight and record the angle at which pain is felt. This is a test for nerve root irritability or dural irritability. A positive result may be shown by back pain or leg pain or both. True sciatica is pain in the buttock and back of the leg, sometimes to the foot, and is usually aggravated by straight leg raising.

Perform a brief neurological examination. Try to think of patterns of abnormality rather than just examining everything.

Prolapsed intervertebral discs occur in the lower lumbar spine mainly and if accompanied by symptoms and signs in the legs, give rise to certain patterns:

L5-S1 prolapse (S1 root compression)
— Depressed ankle jerk. Loss of sensation in the outer side of the sole of the foot. Power loss is unusual and difficult to elicit clinically.

L4-5 prolapse (L5 root compression)
— There is no reflex involved. Weakness occurs in dorsiflexion and eversion. The first muscle to be involved is extensor hallucis longus. Test the power of extension of the hallux. Loss of sensation may be noticed on the outer aspect of the lower leg and the medial aspect of the sole.

L3-4 prolapse (L4 root compression)
— There may be quadriceps weakness and depression or absence of the knee jerk. Sensory changes are often difficult to elicit and unreliable.

Test the plantar responses.

Feel the peripheral pulses.

After all this a general examination should be performed. Examine thyroid, chest, abdomen, breasts and prostate gland where appropriate. As a general rule it is advisable to examine the prostate in males over 50 years of age.

The initial examination is completed by taking relevant radiographs. The standard X-rays are anteroposterior and lateral films, usually with the pelvis. Many clinicians choose to have oblique films if the lumbar spine is involved.

EXAMINATION OF THE KNEE — SPECIAL FEATURES

History

The knee joint gives rise to some typical symptoms. In addition to enquiries about pain and swelling the clinician must ask particularly about the following:

    History of trauma
    Giving way
    Locking
    Clicking and sensation of abnormal movement

Internal derangements of the knee are common. A story of an injury particularly while weight bearing and twisting followed by episodes of pain, swelling, giving way and locking is highly suggestive of an internal derangement or ligament damage leading to collateral or rotatory instability. The knee joint is frequently involved in polyarthritic diseases.

Examination

As hip disease frequently manifests by pain felt in the knee, a brief examination of the hip joint must be performed to exclude this referred pain.

The knee joint is inspected and palpated in the ordinary way. Quadriceps wasting is usually present in knee disorders (especially vastus medialis) and an effusion can often be demonstrated.

Movements must be tested (passive movements are more useful). Note that loss of hyperextension compared with that of the normal side is an important sign. It is convenient to record movements of up to 100° of flexion by measurement but after this it may be more effective to measure the buttock—heel distance of both legs on full flexion for clinical records. An inability to achieve full active extension where passive extension is full is called an extension lag and indicates a failure in the extensor mechanism.

The collateral stability is tested by stressing the joint when it is in a few degrees of flexion. The cruciate ligaments are tested by flexing the knee and drawing the tibia forward or pushing it backwards on the femur. More sophisticated clinical tests are required to demonstrate rotatory instability but they need not concern the undergraduate student.

The joint lines are palpated for tenderness.

The borders of the patella are palpated for tenderness. An additional test for patellar pain is to grind the patella across the underlying femur. Pain and crepitus in the region of the patella during flexion and extension often indicates patello-femoral compartment disease.

Examination of the patella should include observation of the 'tracking' during movement, undue laxity and also patellar apprehension. This refers to a test for potential lateral dislocation of the patella. The patella is pushed laterally while the knee is flexed and extended. The patient feels discomfort and a physical sensation of impending dislocation — 'patellar apprehension'.

Many surgeons choose to test the knee for abnormal clicks or clunks by flexing and extending the knee when internal and external rotation forces are applied to the tibia. One of the manoeuvres is traditionally named the McMurray test. When positive these tests may indicate a tear of a meniscus. However, they are not consistently of great value.

Radiography should include A-P and lateral films and tunnel and skyline views to show all the joint surfaces.

Special investigations include contrast medium/air arthrography and also arthroscopy.

Arthritis

The term arthritis refers to inflammation of a joint. It is commonly used to describe both inflammatory conditions and degenerative disease.

Osteoarthrosis (osteoarthritis) is traditionally regarded as monoarticular (which it often isn't) and the inflammatory arthritides and crystal deposition diseases as polyarticular.

OSTEOARTHROSIS (osteoarthritis)

This is a degenerative disease of joints, a wear and tear arthritis which is primarily a disease of articular cartilage and subchondral bone. There is cartilage and bone destruction, attempts at repair and secondary inflammation, fibrosis and contracture in the synovium and joint capsule.

Aetiology

Although in many cases no explanation for the disease is apparent (Primary Osteoarthrosis) in most cases a predisposing cause may be evident (Secondary Osteoarthrosis) if looked for carefully.

Any disease which damages a joint will predispose it to osteoarthrosis. This might be congenital deformity, trauma, infection, inflammatory arthritis, crystal deposition disease etc.

Pathology

The first changes are in the articular cartilage which loses the outer zone of matrix, becomes fibrillated and split and erosions gradually lead to loss of cartilage and exposure and eburnation of the underlying bone.

The subchondral bone plate is sclerosed in places and replaced by cysts and vascular connective tissue in others. Attempts at repair create fibrocartilage and osteocartilaginous outgrowths — osteophytes. The

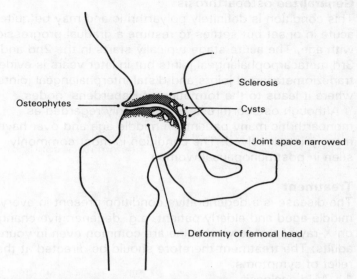

Fig. 31 Radiological features of osteoarthrosis of the hip.

synovium becomes chronically inflamed due to the accumulation of debris leading to capsular fibrosis, contracture and deformity.

Radiological appearances

With the pathology freshly in mind it is quite simple to construct a mental picture of the radiological appearances of osteoarthrosis (Fig. 31).

1. Diminution of joint space
2. Subchondral sclerosis and bone cysts
3. Osteophyte formation
4. Deformity
5. Evidence of underlying disease

Clinical features

Pain
Stiffness
Deformity
Signs of inflammation (usually low grade but exacerbations occur)
Crepitus
Limp

Generalized osteoarthrosis

This condition is definitely polyarthritic and may be quite acute in onset but settles to resume a gradual progression with age. The acute stage typically starts in the 2nd and 3rd metacarpophalangeal joints but in later years is evident in trapeziometacarpal joints and distal interphalangeal joints where it leads to the formation of Heberdens' nodes.

Although osteoarthrosis is commonly regarded as monoarthritic many patients in middle age and over have many joints involved. The condition is most commonly seen in postmenopausal women.

Treatment

The disease is a degenerative condition present in every middle-aged and elderly patient, e.g. degenerative changes on X-ray of the cervical spine are common even in young adults. The treatment therefore should be directed at the relief of symptoms:

1. Mild analgesia
2. Non-steroidal anti-inflammatory drugs, e.g. indomethacin
3. Simple aids, e.g. walking stick, shoe raise
4. Physiotherapy
5. Reduction of activity, e.g. retirement from heavy job
6. Surgery

Surgery in osteoarthritis

The place of surgery can best be shown on a diagram (Fig. 32). The operations available are:

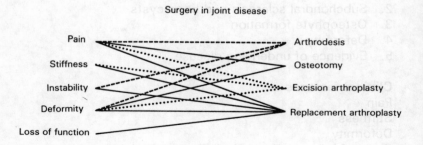

Surgery in joint disease

Pain
Stiffness
Instability
Deformity
Loss of function

Arthrodesis
Osteotomy
Excision arthroplasty
Replacement arthroplasty

Fig. 32   Note that replacement arthroplasty achieves all the targets.

1. Arthrodesis — surgical fusion of a joint.
2. Osteotomy — an operation to divide a bone near a joint to alter the mechanics of weight bearing and to alter the blood supply. The mechanism of pain relief is ill understood.
3. Excision Arthroplasty — the joint is excised and a pseudoarthrosis formed.
4. Replacement arthroplasty — an artificial joint is inserted.

On occasions a surgical 'tidying' of a joint, removing debris, loose bodies and trimming osteophytes may be required.

The symptoms to be relieved are pain, stiffness, instability, deformity and Figure 32 shows which operation helps which symptom.

The polyarthritides

These may be briefly classified as follows:
1. Seropositive polyarthritis — rheumatoid arthritis
2. Seronegative polyarthritis
   a. Seronegative rheumatoid arthritis
   b. Psoriatic arthropathy
   c. Reiter's syndrome
   d. Arthropathy associated with chronic bowel disease
   e. Ankylosing spondylitis
   f. Hypertrophic pulmonary osteoarthropathy
   g. Still's disease
3. Viral polyarthritis
4. Crystal synovitis
   — Gout
   — Pseudogout
5. System diseases
   — Systemic lupus erythematosus.
   — Polyarteritis nodosa
   — Systemic sclerosis
6. Rheumatic fever

RHEUMATOID ARTHRITIS

This is a polyarthritis of uncertain aetiology. It is a systemic connective tissue disorder with mild constitutional symptoms.

The onset may be initiated by infections. Mediated by lysosomal hydrolase the arthritis is promoted by secondary immunological changes, circulatory antibodies, immune complex alterations and cell-mediated hypersensitivity.

Pathology
Synovitis with chronic inflammatory changes.

Synovial hyperplasia leads to invasion and erosion of articular cartilage and subchondral bone. A 'pannus' spreads across the joint. Ultimately the joint is destroyed with ankylosis, deformity or instability resulting. Muscle wasting is associated.

Diagnosis
The student is asked to remember that rheumatoid arthritis is a generalized disease. Constitutional symptoms may be present and other organs involved. These include:
    Vasculitis
    Ocular manifestations
    Splenomegaly and lymphadenopathy
    Pulmonary changes
    Pericarditis
    Anaemia
    Amyloidosis
However, the disease usually presents as a polyarthropathy commencing in the small joints of the hands and feet of young or middle-aged adults. Females are three times as commonly affected as men.

Many other joints may be involved but the disease tends to be peripheral. Soft tissue swelling of joints and morning stiffness are important diagnostic features. When the disease is advanced, the abnormal joints develop characteristic deformities, particularly the hands where joint subluxation, stiffness of the fingers and ulnar drift of the fingers are common. Rheumatoid nodules may be present in the subcutaneous tissues (Fig. 47).

Radiological changes
Initially osteoporosis and soft tissue swelling is noticeable but later erosions appear and progress to subluxation and loss of joint space. Ultimately the joint will be destroyed.

Special investigations

Blood
Anaemia and a raised ESR are common. Tests for
rheumatoid factor are positive in 80% of cases.

Changes in immunoglobulins and positive antinuclear
antibodies sometimes occur.

Synovial fluid
Examine for rheumatoid factor and abnormal (RA) cells.

Synovial biopsy
This is occasionally required if diagnosis is uncertain.

Treatment
The treatment of rheumatoid arthritis is constantly
changing and considerable experience is required to obtain
the best results:
1. Non-steroidal anti-inflammatory drugs:
    Aspirin
    Propionic acids
    Acetic acids
    Ferramic acids
    Enolic acids
2. Steroidal drugs. These should be avoided if possible and
    never used for long periods.
3. Long-acting 'metabolic' drugs:
    Penicillamine
    Gold
    Chloroquine
4. Intra-articular injections of steroids may be useful.
5. During active phases patients may need to be admitted
    for rest, for splinting of joints, physiotherapy etc. They
    will need reassurance, support and possibly aids to daily
    living. The whole patient must be treated and
    consideration given to family and employment.
6. Surgery. The general principles already discussed under
    'Osteoarthrosis' apply here. However, there is
    sometimes a place for prophylactic surgery —
    synovectomy to arrest disease in individual joints and to
    protect tendons from attrition rupture. The surgery of
    rheumatoid arthritis is varied and complex and not within
    the scope of this small book.

THE SERONEGATIVE POLYARTHRITIDES

These have certain clinical differences from rheumatoid arthritis.
1. They are seronegative.
2. They may have central joints involved, particularly the sacro-iliac joint.
3. They may involve distal interphalangeal joints which is uncommon in rheumatoid arthritis.

Psoriatic arthropathy
Occurs in a proportion of psoriatic patients. Beware, the disease may be only visible on the scalp or in nail changes, e.g. pitting.

Reiter's syndrome
This is a polyarthritis associated with urethritis and conjunctivitis or iridocyclitis. It is sometimes a sexually transmitted disease, but may occur in other circumstances such as intestinal inflammation.

Ankylosing spondylitis
This is an arthritis affecting males in early adult life. It commences in the sacro-iliac joints and progresses to the spine producing pain, stiffness and increasing deformity. The patient becomes progressively bent forward and the chest expansion decreases.

   The anterior longitudinal ligaments ossify, producing the well known 'bamboo spine'. This ossification together with sacro-iliitis is visible on radiographs.

Hypertrophic pulmonary osteoarthropathy
This condition occurs in patients with pulmonary disease (usually carcinoma of the bronchus) and is characterized by clubbing and radiological signs of periostitis near the affected joints.

Still's disease
This seronegative polyarthritis occurs in children. There are definite associated constitutional symptoms, fever, rash, lymphadenopathy, hepatosplenomegaly etc. Nodules are

rare. Major joints such as the sacro-iliac joints are commonly affected.

CRYSTAL SYNOVITIS
Gout
This is an inborn error of purine metabolism resulting in diminished excretion of uric acid. It affects middle-aged and elderly males. Traditionally linked with rich foods the attacks are in fact more likely to be provoked by alcohol excess or to follow trauma or surgery.

Uric acid is deposited as crystals of sodium bi-urate. The crystals may be intra-articular, peri-articular or into soft tissues elsewhere, bursae and fascial planes.

Typically the acute attack occurs in the metatarso-phalangeal joint of the great toe which becomes acutely inflamed and painful. However, orthopaedic surgeons frequently see this condition masquerading as an acute infection of a joint or even in extra articular tissues.

In chronic gout widespread deposits occur with gouty deposits called tophi in such sites as earlobe and olecranon bursa. Ultimately widespread joint destruction may occur. Radiographs may show bone erosions adjacent to joints.

Two investigations are helpful: (1) The serum uric acid may be raised. (2) Polarized light microscopy of joint aspirate may show typical birefringent crystals.

Treatment of acute gout is by prescription of the more powerful non-steroidal anti-inflammatory drugs or colchicine.

Chronic gout or persisting high serum uric acid levels may require long-term therapy with probenecid or allopurinol.

Pseudogout (Pyrophosphate deposition disease)
In this condition pyrophosphate crystals showing negative birefringence to polarized light are deposited in joints. Clinically the condition usually presents as an acute arthritis in one large joint.

The condition is one of the causes of chondrocalcinosis. X-rays show calcification of menisci and articular cartilage in joints. In the long term considerable joint destruction may result.

Treatment of acute attacks is much the same as that of acute gout, with such drugs as indomethacin.

MISCELLANEOUS CONDITIONS OF JOINTS

Haemophilia and other coagulation disorders

Repeated haemorrhages into joints result in degenerative changes, capsular fibrosis, contracture and deformity.

Treatment is preventive with active management of acute episodes with antihaemophilic factor (Factor VIII).

Neuropathic joints

In patients with diseases which reduce pain, sensation and proprioceptive perception, joints may become rapidly destroyed by what is an exaggeration of wear and tear.

The diagnosis is suggested by the absence or mildness of pain, the bizarre appearance of destructive changes on the radiographs and evidence of neurological disorder. Typical conditions producing neuropathic joints are syphilis or syringomyelia.

Osteochondritis dissecans

This is a condition in childhood usually affecting the knee in which an osteochondral fragment of bone becomes avascular, loosens and drops away to form a loose body. Symptoms are mild initially but once the fragment is loose the typical features of a loose body in the joint may appear.

The condition is diagnosed radiologically with the 'loose' fragment usually visible in the typical position on the lateral aspect of the medial femoral condyle (Fig. 33).

The condition is less commonly seen in other joints.

Loose bodies

The student is asked not to refer to loose bodies as 'foreign bodies', a common error.

Loose bodies in joints are associated with a typical symptom pattern:

    Episodes of pain and swelling
    Episodes of locking
    Episodes of giving way.

Sometimes the patient becomes aware of the loose body and can manipulate it — a 'joint mouse'.

Causes of loose bodies are as follows:
1.   Trauma — osteochondral fracture.
2.   Degenerative or inflammatory diseases — fibrous,

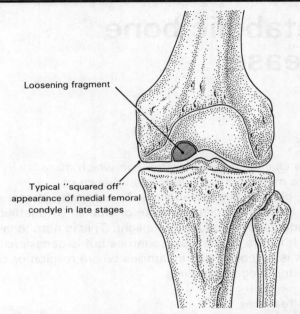

Loosening fragment

Typical "squared off" appearance of medial femoral condyle in late stages

Fig. 33 Osteochondritis dissecans of the knee. Note the typical site on the lateral aspect of the medial femoral condyle.

cartilaginous or osteochondral debris may form a loose body.

3. Osteochondritis dissecans — as above.
4. Synovial Osteochondromatosis — a condition in which cartilaginous nodules are produced in the synovium.

Pigmented villonodular synovitis

This odd condition is a chronic monoarticular proliferative inflammatory reaction characterized by thickening and shagginess of the synovium into which haemosiderin is deposited staining the synovium a dark red-brown colour.

The condition may produce a chronic synovitis, it may erode adjacent bone in a scalloped fashion or form soft tissue masses near joints which are a diagnostic puzzle.

Metabolic bone disease

RICKETS

This is a disease of growing bone in which there is defective mineralization due to disturbance of calcium—phosphorus metabolism. The majority of cases are due to deficient dietary intake of vitamin D together with inadequate exposure to sunlight. This is nutritional rickets. It is rare in Western countries but is occasionally seen (as is osteomalacia) in families where religion or culture dictate strict vegetarian diets.

Clinical features
1. In early infancy hypocalcaemia may result in tetany or convulsions.
2. The older child shows a prominent forehead, retarded growth, bowing of long bones, enlarged epiphyses and deformity of the rib cage.
3. Radiography shows widening and 'cupping' of epiphyses. The wrist joint is usually selected where the distal end of the radius shows the changes well.
4. Serum phosphate level and serum calcium/phosphate ratio are lowered and serum alkaline phosphatase raised.
   Note: Other forms of rickets do occur as a result of hereditary disorders, renal disease, coeliac disease or the administration of anticonvulsant drugs.

Treatment
Treatment with vitamin D cures the disease.
   Orthopaedic surgery may be required if deformities are severe.

OSTEOMALACIA AND OSTEOPOROSIS

Osteomalacia is really adult rickets and is usually of the nutritional type. Although young adults, usually Asians on vegetarian diets, may occasionally acquire the disease, it is more commonly found in elderly patients who neglect their diet.

Because osteomalacia is so closely linked with osteoporosis clinically, it is proposed to discuss the two diseases together. Elderly patients often have thinner and weaker bones and are thus more prone to skeletal injury. In this sense such fractures may be regarded as pathological.

Osteomalacia is a condition in which there is an inadequate amount of calcium or phosphorus or both for mineralization of osteoid which is formed to replace bone lost by normal catabolic lysis. In adults the disease may be caused by deficiencies in absorption of calcium or vitamin D from the bowel or excessive loss of serum phosphorus from the kidneys. It is essentially a disease of mineralization and there is no interference with organic matrix formation (cf. osteoporosis in which there is a deficiency of organic matrix formation). As has been explained the two conditions may coexist.

The disease may be associated with bone pain, pathological fractures and even bone deformity. However, the full-blown picture is rare in the Western hemisphere. Milder degrees are, however, quite common and the condition should be borne in mind in elderly patients with fractures particularly if the fractures are repeated or fail to heal. Radiographs may be difficult to distinguish from those of osteoporotic patients. The bones are more radiolucent than normal, the trabecular pattern may be coarser and focal areas of radiolucency called pseudofractures or Looser's zones may be present. Later the cortices become thinner and less opaque and finally bone deformity and pathological fracture may be seen. The serum calcium or the calcium phosphate ratio may be below normal and the serum alkaline phosphatase is raised. In the last resort the condition may be diagnosed by bone biopsy.

There are many causes for osteoporosis but the common variety affecting old people is due to the hormonal changes of later life particularly in postmenopausal women. It is well known that oestrogen and androgen levels or a combination of the two influence osteoblastic activity. Osteoporosis is the result of failure in the production of adequate amounts of organic bone matrix, osteoid.

Histologically, osteoporotic bones show thinning of the compacta and widening of the Haversian canals. The trabeculae of cancellous tissue are thin and often distorted by fractures. The ratio of bone mass to medullary soft tissue is greatly decreased and there are considerably fewer osteoblasts than in normal bone.

Radiologically osteoporotic bones show greater translucency than normal. The cortices are thin and trabeculae fine and rather sparse. There may be pathological fractures such as the commonly seen compression fractures of vertebrae.

The osteoporosis of the elderly may be worsened by disuse atrophy particularly if these patients are confined to bed for a few weeks. Poor teeth or general disinterest in preparing food may result in a diet deficient in protein, calorie intake, calcium and vitamin D so that osteomalacia may add to the weakening of the osteoporotic bones.

Treatment of osteomalacia and osteoporosis
Osteomalacia responds well to therapy with calcium supplements and vitamin D.

Osteoporosis is a much more difficult problem. It may well be that prolonged hormone replacement therapy with calcium supplements at the time of the menopause may prevent this condition — this is not as yet proven. Once bone loss is established it is probably not possible to replace it. Treatment with calcium and anabolic steroids may prevent further deterioration. Orthopaedic surgery may be necessary to treat the complications.

HYPERPARATHYROIDISM

This is a condition caused by excessive secretion of parathormone by hyperplasia or more usually an adenoma of the parathyroid gland.

Diagnosis
1. Dyspepsia, malaise, vomiting, weakess, polyuria.
2. Demineralization of bone, bone pain, bone cysts and deformity.
3. Calcification and stone formation in kidneys.
4. Radiographs show generalized demineralization, bone

'cysts' and subperiosteal erosions.
5. Serum calcium is raised.
6. Urinary calcium excretion is raised.

Treatment is by excision of the adenoma.

PAGET'S DISEASE

Although this is strictly not a metabolic disease, it is convenient to include it in this chapter.

Paget's disease is a condition of bone of unknown aetiology. Bone turnover is altered. The trabeculae become coarser and fewer in number and the bones more spongy, broader and weaker. Bending and fractures are common.

Clinical features
1. The majority of cases are symptomless and merely accidental findings on radiographs taken for other purposes.
2. Bone pain occurs in more severe cases.
3. Enlargement of the skull, deformity of long bones particularly the tibia. Pathological fractures occur.
4. Cranial nerve lesions may accompany skull enlargement.
5. High output cardiac failure may result in severe cases.

Treatment
In severe cases calcitonin or diphosphonates may be used. Mild cases require no treatment.

Infections of bone and joint

When the word 'infection' is mentioned the student should immediately subdivide his or her thoughts as follows:

Infection — Acute
            — Chronic — Specific
                        — Non-specific

ACUTE INFECTION OF BONE AND JOINT

Bacteriology

The great majority of acute infections of bone and joint are caused by *Staphylococcus aureus*.

Following far behind in frequency is a miscellany of organisms occasionally encountered.

Streptococci
Haemophilus influenzae
Pneumococci
E. coli
Gonococci
Salmonellae
Brucellae

It is stated that sickle cell disease predisposes the patient to bone infection caused by salmonellae. It is probable, however, that the disease predisposes the patient to bone infection and the organisms vary in prevalence in different parts of the world.

Who gets these conditions?

The majority of sufferers are babies and young children. Both sexes are affected. The diseases fall into two main groups:

1. The 'typical' involving infants and young children and showing the classic features.
2. The 'atypical' presentations of the neonatal period.
   These will be discussed in more detail later.

Which bones or joints are most affected?

In orthopaedics things tend to happen near the knee. Infections are no exception. Osteitis is commonest at the upper tibia or lower femur and acute pyogenic arthritis at the knee or hip. However, other bones and other joints may be affected.

Infections of the spine

These need special mention as they show certain characteristics of their own.

1 Unusual site

The infections occur usually in the disc space eroding adjacent bone. Compare this with the disc preservation shown on radiographs of other conditions of the spine (Fig. 1, p. 4).

2 Presentation

Although infections in the spine may present acutely it is more common for them to run a 'chronic' course despite the presence of organisms which behave 'acutely' at other sites.

Pathogenesis of acute infections

The majority of infections of bone or joint are caused by blood-borne organisms arising in the upper respiratory tract, tooth sockets etc.

Joints, however, have a joint cavity with walls which are in part made up of adjacent bones. Therefore it is possible for joints to be infected by penetration from without and by extension of infection from adjacent bone.

Note that it is unusual in the older infant or child to find extension of infection from the metaphysis of the bone across the epiphyseal plate. In the neonatal period, however, this does occur.

The natural history of 'typical' acute osteitis

The infection occurs in the metaphysis of the bone. Supplying the adjacent epiphyseal plate are arcades of capillaries and it is thought that slowing of flow in these capillaries allows circulating organisms to settle.

We now have a bone abscess and it is at this stage that we have to diagnose and to treat successfully any such infection. The pus does not usually cross the epiphyseal plate but may track down the shaft (diaphysis) and also outwards to form a subperiosteal abscess (Fig. 34).

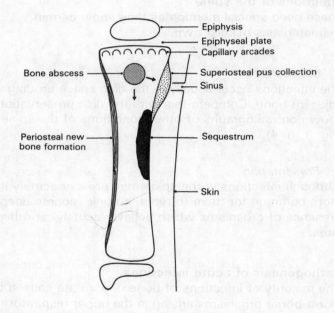

Fig. 34 The natural history of acute osteomyelitis.

The stimulated periosteum lays down new bone (involucrum). The combination of bacterial toxins, enzymes, raised pressure, thrombosis of veins and stripping of periosteum may result in death of sections of bone. These are called sequestra.

Eventually the infection may burst out to form a sinus discharging pus and fragments of dead bone. Retrograde colonization of the sinuses with mixed flora from without ensures chronicity. This is the stage of chronic osteomyelitis.

In rare cases persisting chronic infection may even lead to amyloid disease.

Clinical presentation of 'typical' acute osteitis
   Signs of pus general
   Signs of pus local
   PAIN
   The patient will show general signs of acute infection
with pyrexia, malaise and in some cases profound toxaemia.
   Locally PAIN predominates. These infections are very
painful and the patient may be fearful of any movement or
examination. Heat, redness, swelling, tenderness and loss
of function are usually all apparent. These are the classic
signs of inflammation.

The natural history of acute pyogenic arthritis
A blood-borne infection settles in the synovial lining of a
joint and the joint cavity becomes infected (synovitis). By
transudate and exudate a joint effusion develops. The
effusion is an excellent culture medium. (Hence the need to
drain infected joints early.)
   Organisms proliferate and produce toxins and enzymes.
Added to these are proteases arising from the destruction of
neutrophils. The articular cartilage is vulnerable to attack
by proteases, fibrinolysins and hyaluronidase and will be
rapidly destroyed. If untreated, the joint destruction
continues. Fibrous and even bony ankylosis may occur and
sinuses form.
   It must be apparent that successful treatment depends
upon overcoming the infection before articular cartilage
damage occurs.

Clinical presentation of 'typical' acute pyogenic arthritis
   Signs of pus general
   Signs of pus local
   Signs associated with the presence of a joint cavity
   PAIN
   In addition to the general and local features of pus, joint
infections have certain additional features.
   The joint cavity will show swelling and effusion.
   The joint will adopt a position of maximum capacity
(usually flexion) and sometimes muscle spasm may dictate
position.
   Note that although muscle wasting is a typical finding in
chronic inflammation of a joint, there is not time for this to
develop in the initial phases of acute infections.

Special investigations
1. The white blood count may be raised.
2. The erythrocyte sedimentation rate is raised.
3. A blood culture may grow the infecting organism in about half the cases.
4. If a joint is involved it may be aspirated immediately. Microscopy of the aspirate will often suggest which organism is involved. Culture of the aspirate will identify the organism subsequently and antibiotic sensitivities will become available to the clinician.
5. In cases with a longer history it may be possible to demonstrate antistaphylococcal antibodies.

X-ray examination
This is usually of little value in the early stages. Soft tissue swelling or an increase in joint space may be visible but no bony changes will appear early.

At about 10 days after the onset of infection, X-ray changes appear. Periosteal new bone formation plus an osteolytic lesion in the metaphysis is the typical appearance of acute osteitis at this later stage. Osteoporosis and joint space narrowing may be a late feature of pyogenic arthritis.

Treatment of acute infections of bone and joint
Rest — general
Rest — local
Antibiotics
Surgical drainage
The child will usually take to his bed or cot himself.
Local rest can be achieved by splinting. It is preferable to use a splint which does not obscure the affected bone so that regular observations may be made of progress.

Antibiotics
It is customary to make an assumption that the infection is staphylococcal until proved otherwise.

Appropriate antibiotics must be given in large doses and preferably intravenously in the first instance.

Fucidic acid plus flucloxacillin or fucidic acid plus erythromycin are favoured combinations.

After the infection has settled initially, the antibiotic therapy may be changed to 'oral' administration but it should be continued for approximately six weeks. Naturally the clinician will be guided by clinical response, sedimentation rate etc.

Surgical drainage
There are two main indications for surgical intervention in any disease, anywhere in the body. These are:
1.   Unsuitability for non-surgical treatment.
2.   Failure of non-surgical treatment.
   In the case of acute pyogenic infections of joints we have already noted the urgency to drain the joint and to prevent articular cartilage damage. Thus we can state that infected joints are not suitable for non-surgical treatment and early drainage is essential.
   On the other hand acute pyogenic osteitis often responds well to conservative treatment and surgical drainage may not be required. The progress of the disease is watched. If after 36 hours there is no general or local improvement then surgical drainage is indicated. Surgical drainage of a bone is usually performed by drilling holes in the bone at intervals starting in the metaphysis and continuing in the direction of the diaphysis until no further pus escapes.

The 'atypical' presentation of acute pyogenic osteitis and arthritis in the neonatal period
There are considerable differences between infections in the neonatal period and those in older babies and children. Beware of the unusual!
1.   Unusual organisms may be encountered.
2.   The bone or joint infection may be masked by generalized septicaemia. Florid local signs of infection may be absent, particularly if the septicaemia has been vigorously treated by intravenous antibiotics.
3.   Infection with unusual organisms may lead to very 'quiet' infections. Often the only physical sign is unwillingness to move the limb. Beware of low-grade infections of the hip joint. It may be preferable to risk a negative exploration than to allow a hip joint to be destroyed through overcautiousness.
4.   The epiphysis is not a barrier to infection in this age

group. Combined osteitis and pyogenic arthritis may occur.

CHRONIC INFECTIONS OF BONE AND JOINT

We have already mentally divided infections into specific and non-specific. What does this mean?

Non-specific chronic infections are those in which an organism normally associated with an acute infection presents in a chronic fashion.

1. We have already noted that this may occur in infection of the intervertebral disc space (discitis).
2. The other classic example is the Brodie's Abscess. This is a chronic abscess of bone, usually near the metaphysis which develops without any acute illness. It is characterized by deep boring pain in the bone and is usually diagnosed when the relevant bone is X-rayed. A radiolucent area surrounded by a zone of sclerosis is typical.

Specific chronic infections are those caused by an organism which usually gives rise to a chronic illness. Tuberculosis is by far the most important but a simplified list of these is as follows:

Tuberculosis
Spirochaetal infection — Syphilis
                        — Yaws
Actinomycosis
Tropical fungi

Tuberculosis of bone and joint

Epidemiology
Tuberculosis is a chronic infection caused by *Mycobacterium tuberculosis*. It occurs worldwide particularly in the Third World. In European countries it is more common in immigrants from the 'third world' than in the indigenous population. Bone and joint disease occurs in about 5% of all cases and the infection is divided approximately equally between spinal infection and infection of major joints.

The infective nature of the disease and the higher incidence in certain groups of people make the taking of a family history or other history of exposure to the disease an important part of the diagnosis.

Pathology
Tuberculosis of bone and joint is a blood-borne infection which may be conveniently thought of as 'metastatic' disease. The primary site is nearly always the lung. The victim has usually already suffered a primary infection and shows immune and hypersensitivity responses.

Some organs are remarkably resistant to 'metastatic' infection but infection of others, particularly the urogenital system, is common and should be looked for.

The disease is characterized by a typical inflammatory reaction, bone destruction and replacement with granulation tissue. Tuberculous abscesses, pus tracking between tissue planes and sinus formation are common.

Large joints initially suffer a synovitis which progresses slowly to joint destruction and erosion of adjacent bone.

Spinal tuberculosis typically arises in a disc space but may also arise in the vertebral body itself and 'skip' lesions are not uncommon. Bone destruction causes collapse anteriorly and an angular kyphosis or gibbus posteriorly. Paraverterbal abscesses may occur. The tuberculous pus may track to present as 'cold' abscess some distance away, e.g. Psoas abscess. Here the pus has tracked down the psoas muscle to present as a cold abscess in the groin. A paraparesis of gradual onset may be caused by local pressure, local pachymeningitis or vascular impairment.

A more rare and curious presentation of bone tuberculosis is tuberculous dactylitis. Here a phalanx or metacarpal develops a fusiform swelling which later shows bone destruction and periosteal new bone formation.

Diagnosis of tuberculosis of bone and joint
    History of contact
    Signs of tuberculosis general
    Signs of tuberculosis local
    Radiological changes
    Special investigations
The patient may have a history of contact or he is in an 'at risk' community. There may be malaise, loss of weight, and night sweats. There may be local pain, stiffness or limping.

Local signs of inflammation in major joints may be conveniently thought of as similar to those in acute infections but much less dramatic and slower in onset. In addition muscle wasting will be a dramatic feature. As the infection progresses slowly the position of joints adapting to position of maximum capacity or to muscle spasm may be noticeable. (Low grade synovitis, local warmth and swelling, cold abscesses, deformity of spine, or other bones or joints are typical features.)

Radiography
Radiographs in the early stages may show local osteoporosis around joints with soft tissue swelling and increased joint space. Later, evidence of destruction and joint space narrowing occur.

The typical anterior bone collapse of vertebrae may be present and paravertebral abscesses seen.

The chest X-ray may show the initial pulmonary infection.

Special investigations
1. Blood count and ESR.
2. Mantoux test — this is a skin test for hypersensitivity reactions. Whereas a negative result strongly suggests that tuberculosis is not the cause, a positive result is less useful.
3. Microscopy and culture of synovial fluid or pus. Ziehl–Nielsen staining may show acid-fast bacilli. Unfortunately culture of the bacilli is slow and a bacteriological confirmation of the diagnosis may take three weeks or more.
4. Biopsy by needle or open operation should be performed in all cases where diagnosis is uncertain, particularly in countries where tuberculosis is uncommon. Biopsy may be of bone or synovium.
5. A search should be made for 'metastatic' disease elsewhere. At the very least the urine should be examined for the 'sterile' pyuria which typifies tuberculosis of the urinary tract.
6. In cases where confirmation of diagnosis proves difficult, it is quite respectable to institute a therapeutic trial with antibiotic therapy.

Treatment
   Rest — general
   Rest — local
   Antituberculous therapy
   Surgical intervention
   Attention to nutrition and rest is important and local splinting of the diseased joint is advantageous in the early more acute phases. The main treatment, however, is by antituberculous therapy. The favoured regime at present is to use rifampicin plus isonicotinic acid hydrazide (Isoniazid) for 12–18 months. Note the necessity for prolonged treatment and follow up. Streptomycin and para-aminosalicylic acid are used less frequently but are inexpensive and there are other drugs available if resistant organisms are encountered.

Surgical intervention
1. Drainage of abscesses.
2. Excision of diseased bone sometimes with primary bone grafting as is sometimes advocated in spinal tuberculosis.
3. Decompression and fusion if paraplegia is present.
4. Synovectomy in selected cases.
5. Salvage procedures including correction of deformities and arthrodesis of diseased joints.
   Note that surgery is always performed under cover of antituberculous drugs.

Bone tumours

The student must be able to repeat one of the standard definitions of a neoplasm.

A neoplasm is a growth of new cells. This growth is unco-ordinated with that of normal tissue.

In these cells there is a loss of control of reproduction and differentiation.

The growth continues after the cessation of the stimulus which provoked it.

PERSPECTIVE

Secondary malignant tumours of bone are very much more common than primary malignant tumours. It is said that primary malignant tumours of bone number less than 1% of all primary malignancies.

However, these primary malignancies attract attention for two reasons. First, they have a very bad prognosis. Secondly they constitute one of the most important groups of primary malignant tumours in patients under twenty years of age.

WHAT IS A HAMARTOMA?

A hamartoma is a congenital malformation of tissues which in some ways resemble a neoplasm. The cells which are present are disorganized in their distribution but behave normally and are cells which can be expected to be found at that site.

The reason for digression at this point is that the common exostosis or osteochondroma is probably more correctly placed in this group. These 'tumours' are capped by epiphyseal cartilage and usually cease to grow when the adjacent epiphysis fuses, i.e. they do respond to cessation of the stimulus to growth.

Osteochondromas are sometimes multiple and are found mainly around the knee, the upper humerus and lower radius. In fact these are also the sites of predilection of many true neoplasms of bone.

CLASSIFICATION OF TUMOURS OF BONE AND ASSOCIATED TISSUES

It is convenient to classify tumours of bone and associated tissues according to their tissue of origin. It is also convenient to give them a 'star rating' so that the student may have an idea of their relative clinical importance and the interest shown in them by examiners. In addition to the named tumours there are many benign bone tumours which attract the attention of specialist orthopaedic surgeons but it is not necessary for the student to know details of them all.

'Star rating' system
The tumours will be 'star rated' on a scale 1–3 (Table 1). The more stars the more important clinically and for the purposes of examination! The student should know something about all 'star rated' tumours.

Table 1

Tissue of origin	Benign tumour	Malignant tumour
Osteoblast	Osteoblastoma	Osteosarcoma***
Osteoclast	Osteoclastoma*	
Chondroblast	Chondroblastoma	Chondrosarcoma**
	Chondroma* (Enchondroma) (Ecchondroma)	
Fibroblast	Fibroma	Fibrosarcoma**
Synovium		Synovial sarcoma**
?		Ewings sarcoma**
Plasma cells		Myeloma**

The 2–3 star tumours have much in common. They are all mesenchymal tumours, sarcomas, and they show the characteristics of that group of tumours. They are very active, locally invasive and metastasize early to the lungs by bloodspread. Only one will be described in detail, but of the others only such information will be given as distinguishes one from another.

Tumours of associated tissues
The mesenchymal cells of bone, cartilage or synovium do not of course exist in isolation. In the marrow cavity are reticulo-endothelial cells and haemopoietic cells. The bone is supported by soft tissue, blood vessels and the periosteum by nerves. All these tissues may develop neoplastic change. Thus we may have:
  Supporting tissue tumours, e.g. angioma, angiosarcoma.
  Reticulo-endothelial tumours, e.g. lymphoma, myeloma.
  'Tumours' of haemopoietic tissue, e.g. leukaemia.

DIAGNOSIS OF BONE TUMOURS

As with any tumour anywhere, the student should think of bone tumours as presenting in two ways:
1. Because they are there   — pain
                              — swelling
2. Because they complicate   — pathological fracture
                              — haemorrhage into joint or
                                soft tissue
                              — metastases
Once attention has been drawn to the bone then radiographs are taken and the lesion revealed (Fig. 35). With experience a radiologist can make a fairly reliable guess at the nature of the lesion but ultimately a biopsy will have to be performed.

HISTOLOGY OF BONE TUMOURS

The histology of bone tumours is very difficult, particularly if a pathological fracture is present. Great expertise is required. No case should commence treatment before an adequate biopsy has been taken. This should include bone and soft tissue.

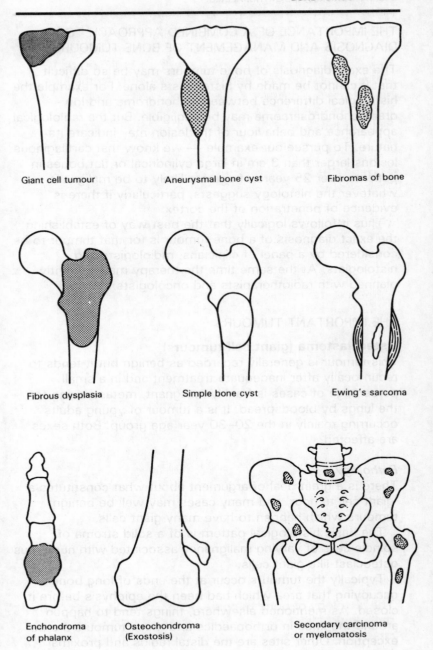

Giant cell tumour   Aneurysmal bone cyst   Fibromas of bone

Fibrous dysplasia   Simple bone cyst   Ewing's sarcoma

Enchondroma   Osteochondroma   Secondary carcinoma
of phalanx   (Exostosis)   or myelomatosis

Fig. 35 Typical radiological appearances of some tumours.

THE IMPORTANCE OF A COMBINED APPROACH TO DIAGNOSIS AND MANAGEMENT OF BONE TUMOURS

The exact diagnosis of bone tumours may be so difficult that it cannot be made by histologists alone. For example the histological difference between a chondroma and low-grade chondrosarcoma may be negligible. But the radiological appearance and behaviour of the lesion may indicate its nature. To pursue our example — we know that cartilaginous lesions larger than 3 cm in large cylindrical or flat bones in patients over 25 years of age are likely to be malignant whatever the histology suggests, particularly if there is evidence of penetration of the cortex.

Thus it follows logically that the best way of establishing the exact diagnosis of a bone tumour is for that tumour to be considered by a panel of clinicians, radiologists and histologists. At the same time the therapy may be jointly planned with radiotherapists and oncologists.

THE IMPORTANT TUMOURS

Osteoclastoma (giant cell tumours)

This tumour is generally regarded as benign but it tends to recur locally after inadequate treatment and in a small percentage of cases is frankly malignant, metastasizing to the lungs by bloodspread. It is a tumour of young adults occurring mainly in the 20–30 year age group. Both sexes are affected.

Pathology

There is a great deal of argument about what constitutes a 'giant cell tumour' and many cases may well be benign tumours which happen to have many giant cells.

The basic histological pattern is of a solid stroma of spindle cells of varying malignancy associated with numerous osteoclast-like giant cells.

Typically the tumours occur at the ends of long bones occupying that area which had been the epiphysis before it closed. As mentioned elsewhere, things tend to happen around the knee in orthopaedics and these tumours are no exception. Other sites are the distal radius and proximal humerus.

The tumours are diagnosed as previously described.

Treatment
Ideally these tumours should be treated with wide local excision even if this means sacrificing a major joint or replacing bone and joint with a 'massive' joint replacement. Curettage and bone grafting is often followed by local recurrence.

Radiotherapy should be reserved for those tumours which are surgically inaccessible.

Chondroma

Clinically these benign tumours present as tumours within bones or enchondromata. Typically the enchondroma is found in a phalanx or metacarpal bone.

Some of these are probably hamartomas and other cartilaginous lesions but it will suffice the student to regard chondroma as an entity.

Chondrosarcoma

This is a malignant tumour of cartilage producing only chondroid and collagen. It is slow growing but ultimately metastasizes by bloodstream to the lungs.

It occurs less commonly than osteosarcoma and in a slightly older age group, 30–50 years. If it is found in younger people it may well have arisen in a pre-existing osteochondroma.

The tumour differs from osteosarcoma in that it occurs approximately equally between the flat bones of the trunk and the round bones of the limbs. It is common around the knee and the proximal ends of femur and humerus. In general the more peripheral a cartilaginous tumour the more likely it is to be benign.

Treatment is by wide excision including amputation if necessary. The prognosis is a little better than osteosarcoma largely because the tumour is slower growing.

Fibrosarcoma of bone

Fibrosarcoma may be endosteal or parosteal. It is much less common than osteosarcoma but occurs in both sexes at the same period of life, the second and third decade. The tumours are slower growing and have a better prognosis than osteosarcoma. Parosteal sarcomas, particularly, may do well with wide local excision with or without chemotherapy.

Synovial sarcoma

These tumours are uncommon but occur in young people most commonly around the knee.

They are characterized by masses of spindle cells plus slit spaces often lined by cells of carcinomatoid type.

Not surprisingly therefore they may metastasize to lymph nodes in addition to the more usual bloodspread to lungs.

Ewing's sarcoma

This is a highly malignant tumour arising in the medulla of bone and probably of myelogenous origin. The cell of origin is not definitely known.

The tumour occurs in young people of both sexes in the second and third decades.

It differs from osteosarcoma in several aspects:
1.   The tumour consists of sheets of round cells.
2.   The tumour may occur in any bone.
3.   The tumour is often found in the middle (diaphysis) of long bones where it excites a marked periosteal reaction.
4.   It may metastasize to other bones in addition to the usual bloodspread to lungs.
5.   The tumour is often accompanied by fever and leucocytosis and is typified by persisting pain.
6.   The prognosis is dreadful and is probably fairly stated as approximately 10% five-year survival.

Osteosarcoma (osteogenic sarcoma)

This is the commonest primary malignant tumour of bone except myeloma. It is very important to the student to know something about this tumour as it has been topical for some years.

The tumour arises from undifferentiated mesenchymal tissue in bone. It arises most commonly in the femur and once again a wave of the hand around the knee will indicate the area of greatest incidence.

The tumour is commonest in the second and third decades of life and affects both sexes, males rather more than females. A second peak occurs later in life in flat bones with an association with Paget's disease.

Pathology
The tumour almost always begins in the metaphysis and grows rapidly destroying the cancellous tissue and often eroding the cortex before diagnosis is made. It bursts out of the cortex forming a soft tissue mass and elevating the periosteum which lays down new bone to form the radiological appearance of Codman's triangle.

The tumour is highly vascular. It consists of a mixture of connective tissue cells but always there will be areas of malignant osteoid. Other cell types are mainly spindle cells and cartilage.

The tumour is locally invasive and metastasizes early by bloodstream to the lungs.

Diagnosis
This is described earlier.

Radiological appearance
The tumour shows mixed areas of osteolysis and osteosclerosis in the metaphysis. It bursts out of the cortex creating a soft tissue mass and provoking the periosteum to lay down new bone. This may give rise to the appearance of Codman's triangle (Fig. 36). Very active new bone formation outside the bone may show as 'sunray' spicules.

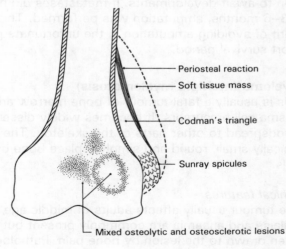

- Periosteal reaction
- Soft tissue mass
- Codman's triangle
- Sunray spicules
- Mixed osteolytic and osteosclerotic lesions

Fig. 36 The 'classical' radiological appearance of osteosarcoma of the distal femur.

Prognosis
This is poor. Some years ago a figure of approximately
20% five-year survival was quoted. With modern methods it
is hoped to improve this to 30–40% five-year survival.
Several multicentric trials are attempting to achieve this kind
of figure.

Treatment
1. Establish diagnosis beyond any reasonable doubt by the
   methods described.
2. Ensure that the patient does not already have pulmonary
   metastases. A chest X-ray is therefore mandatory before
   commencing treatment.
3. Excise the tumour widely. Amputation may be necessary
   but if the tumour is histologically graded as of low
   malignancy, local excision and replacement with a
   'massive' prosthesis may be possible.
4. Commence chemotherapy immediately. Regimes differ
   but the general principle is to use a combination of an
   antimetabolite (e.g. methotrexate) a mustard (e.g.
   chlorambucil) and another cytotoxic substance of
   different method of action.

   An alternative method of treatment now not in vogue,
was to irradiate the primary with large doses of X-rays and
then to await developments. If metastases did not develop
in 3–6 months, amputation was performed. This had the
merit of avoiding amputation in the unfortunate patient's
short survival period.

Myeloma (multiple myelomatosis)
This is usually a fatal tumour of bone marrow arising in
plasma cell precursors. It becomes widely disseminated by
bloodspread to other parts of the skeleton. The lesions are
typically small, round and simply replace bone by plasma
cells.

Clinical features
The tumour usually affects adults of middle age or over.
Malaise and anaemia are commonly present but attention is
often drawn to the lesion by bone pain. Pathological
fractures are common. Radiographs show numerous punched
out translucencies in bone, skull, ribs, pelvis and upper

femur and humerus. These are the areas of active bone marrow. Sometimes the disease is so widespread that the spinal column exhibits an appearance of widespread demineralization.

Typically there is a very high ESR and serum protein electrophoresis shows raised globulin levels.

Marrow biopsy usually confirms diagnosis.

Prognosis
The disease is usually fatal but treatment may prolong life for years.

Treatment
Local lesions may be treated with radiotherapy but the main treatment is by use of cytotoxic agents of the mustard family.

MALIGNANT TUMOURS OF SOFT TISSUE

Fibrosarcoma
This is the commonest malignancy of soft tissues of mesenchymal origin.

Pathology
These are spindle cell tumours of varying malignancy. They may appear encapsulated but spread locally nevertheless. The tumours metastasize late to the lungs.

Clinical features
The tumours present as a slowly enlarging painless mass. They occur at all ages and in both sexes.

Treatment
Wide local excision offers the best hope of cure.

Synovial sarcoma
Discussed previously (p. 150).

TUMOUR-LIKE CONDITIONS OF BONE

Hamartoma of cartilage
Discussed previously (p. 144).

Solitary bone cyst
These cysts occur in the long bones of children and
adolescents. The humerus is the favourite site. The cysts
may become multiloculated and expand the bone evenly in
all directions. They contain clear fluid and the wall is a thin
layer of connective tissue with some giant cells.

The cysts often present by pathological fracture. Small
cysts require no treatment, but large cysts need curetting
and bone grafting to avoid fracture.

Aneurysmal bone cyst
This is a curious, highly vascular lesion of bone
characterized by a 'bulging out' eccentrically on one side of a
bone. The tumours are found at many sites, e.g. long
bones and spine. Accessible tumours should be curetted
and bone grafted and inaccessible tumours may respond
to radiotherapy. The surgeon should expect considerable
bleeding from this vascular lesion.

Fibrous dysplasia
In this condition parts of a single bone (monostotic) or
several bones (polystotic) are replaced by fibrous tissue.
Long bones are most affected, especially the femur.

The condition presents with pain, deformity and
pathological fracture.

The blood chemistry is normal.

Radiographs show an osteolytic lesion of homogeneous
appearance usually expanding the bone, which is often
deformed.

Treatment may be by prophylactic internal fixation. If the
lesion is extending, the whole lesion may need to be excised
and a bone graft performed.

Histiocystosis X and eosinophilic granuloma
Histiocystosis X refers to a group of conditions where
there is an inflammatory proliferation of histiocytes which
tend to 'store' cholesterol.

The group includes types which affect bones plus other
organs but of more interest to the orthopaedic surgeon is the
condition named eosinophilic granuloma. This is usually a
tumour-like solitary lesion of bone. It favours pelvis, skull or
vertebral body but may involve long bones too. The lesion

has to be distinguished from other lytic lesions of bone. Radiographs show a well defined 'hole' in a bone. If a vertebral body is involved, X-rays may show a dramatic collapse. Diagnosis may have to be established by biopsy which shows a 'granuloma' with many histiocytes and eosinophils.

Often no treatment is necessary as the lesion may resolve spontaneously. Surgical curettage or even radiotherapy may on occasions be indicated.

Osteoid osteoma

This is a benign lesion of bone characterized by causing severe, continuous and boring pain. The pain is said to be worse at night and relieved by aspirin.

When sited centrally in bone the lesion may appear osteolytic but near the cortex the lesion produces a characteristic appearance. There is a dense local sclerosis and thickening, in the centre of which is a small translucent zone. This zone is a small area of what appears to be osteoid (nidus).

Treatment is by block excision of the lesion. Success is accompanied by immediate relief of the characteristic pain.

'Osteochondritis'

This is a group of conditions which are historically regarded as similar in aetiology, clinical presentation and radiological appearances. They are widely distributed and extremely 'untidy' if presented to the student as separate items on a regional basis. The author wishes to familiarize the student with these conditions without presenting them as a large number of incomprehensible diseases.

The conditions almost certainly have no common aetiology and no common clinical presentation but do enjoy a similarity of radiological appearances. In addition they are blessed with a series of eponyms round which orthopaedic surgeons (and examiners) like to roll their tongues —hence the popularity!

These obscure diseases affect developing epiphyseal areas in children and adolescents, all presenting with local pain. The diagnosis is confirmed radiologically and the progress of the disease followed radiologically. The affected bone softens and fragments. It looks dense and fragmented on X-ray. It then heals gradually over a period of 2–3 years with or without deformity. In many instances it has the appearance of avascular necrosis. Indeed some of these conditions probably are due to avascular necrosis whereas others are due to trauma and fatigue or stress injuries of bone. If healing results in deformity of a joint, osteoarthrosis in later life must be expected.

The three most important conditions are Scheurmann's disease of the spine, Perthe's disease of the hip and Osgood-Schlatter's disease of the tibial tuberosity. These three are described elsewhere in the book. The student should be familiar with these conditions and their names.

For the remainder it is necessary only to know that they exist. An undergraduate cannot be expected to remember a list of unimportant eponyms:

The lunate bone (Kienbock's Disease)
The os calcis (Sever's Disease)

The tarsal navicular bone (Kohler's disease)
The head of the second metatarsal bone (Freiberg's disease)

The name 'Calves' disease was given to an 'osteochondritis' of a single vertebra. In reality this condition represents eosinophilic granuloma in a vertebral body.

Paediatric orthopaedics

CONGENITAL ABNORMALITIES OF THE NECK

Problems of neck and scapula development
Congenital fusions or deficiencies of cervical vertebrae are often associated with failure of growth or descent of the scapula. The conditions may be unilateral or bilateral but are characterized by a short neck and elevated shoulder. The affected scapula is small and high and relatively immobile. If unilateral the asymmetry is obvious. The names Klippel-Feil Syndrome and Sprengel's shoulder are associated with two presentations of this group of disorders.

Congenital torticollis
In this condition a lateral inclination of the head or torticollis develops as a result of contracture of an abnormal sterno-mastoid muscle. This is probably an infarction and can sometimes be felt as a 'tumour' during early infancy. The head inclines and, if untreated, facial asymmetry and problems with visual horizons may follow. Early correction is therefore desirable.

Most cases respond to sustained physiotherapy and stretching. An established contracture may require surgical division of the sterno-mastoid muscle at its lower end.

Scoliosis
Scoliosis means a lateral curvature of the spine. Why the condition is so important is that many types of scoliosis progress inexorably giving rise to very ugly deformities, embarrassing respiratory function and even causing neurological lesions.

Untreated cases do badly. If treated early the results are usually excellent. Early diagnosis may be difficult and be best achieved by systematic clinical screening during routine school medical examinations.

Scoliosis may be:
1. Postural — e.g. associated with short lower limb.
2. Structural — Here the cause may be neuropathic, myopathic or osteopathic:
   a. Congenital — often a vertebral abnormality and prognosis is poor.
   b. Paralytic   — associated with trunk muscle paralysis.
   c. Infantile   — the curve is typically gradual and long. The prognosis is usually good with spontaneous correction of the deformity.
   d. Adolescent

Typical idiopathic scoliosis
This is the group in which we are most interested. Girls are more often affected than boys.

The curvature begins in childhood or adolescence and progresses until the end of spinal growth. At the apex of the convexity of the curve, the vertebrae are rotated carrying with them transverse processes and ribs. It is this rib 'hump' which produces the ugly hunchback deformity. Hence it follows that lumbar scoliosis is less conspicuous than thoracic scoliosis.

The diagnostic importance of this rotation is that when a patient's spine is inspected in the forward flexed position any such asymmetry or 'hump' will become apparent (Fig. 37).

Diagnosis
The deformity is recognized because it is noticed. Ideally this should be on routine screening at school clinic.

Radiographs confirm the deformity and are also used for measurement of the deformity and monitoring the progress. The standard X-ray for measurement is a standing antero-posterior radiograph.

Treatment
It is not within the scope of this book to go into the details of treatment. The principles are:
1. If the scoliosis is minor and not progressing then it may be watched or the spine braced until skeletal maturity is reached.

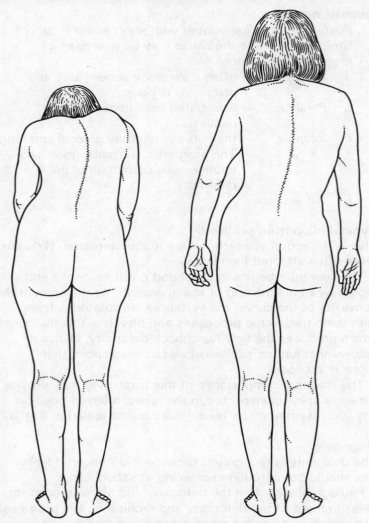

Fig. 37 *Left:* typical idiopathic scoliosis, with a rib hump on bending forward. *Right:* unbalanced or 'total' scoliosis. No rotation would be seen here on flexion.

2.   Curves greater than 40° and any rapidly progressing curve need more active treatment.

3.   The curve is corrected either by external corrective hinged plasters or by internal 'jacking' devices such as Harrington Rods. Having achieved maximum correction then a spinal fusion is performed.

MENINGOMYELOCOELE (spina bifida)

In this condition there is a failure of closure of the neural tube. Induction of mesenchymal tissues making up the spine and the ectodermal tissue of the skin may fail to a greater or lesser extent. Thus we may have spina bifida occulta (where no lesion is apparent on inspection) at one extreme and frank myelomeningocoele at the other.

The student should understand that severe myelomeningocoele is a miserable condition. The natural history is as follows:

1. The child is born with the defect. The exposed neural tissue is vulnerable to mechanical, thermal and chemical trauma and bacterial invasion. Enthusiastic surgery may close the defect by covering it with skin flaps.
2. At about one month hydrocephalus begins. The spinal cord is tethered at the lesion. Differential growth between spinal cord and spinal column pulls the hind brain into the foramen magnum (the Arnold Chiari malformation) and interferes with circulation of cerebrospinal fluid.
3. Paralysed sphincters predispose to recurrent urinary tract infections and urinary diversion may become necessary.
4. The paralysed limbs do not develop and the bones are weak. Pathological fractures are frequent.
5. There is often spinal deformity severe enough to shorten the trunk and interfere with pulmonary function. Recurrent chest infection is common.
6. Obesity may be a problem in children confined to a wheelchair.
7. The child must face up to paralysis, incontinence and impotence. Not surprisingly emotional problems and family disturbances are common.
8. Less than 10% of treated cases may be regarded as 'normal' and many others show evidence of mental deficiency.

Treatment

Much devoted effort has been put into the management of these unfortunate children. Ingenious splinting and aids to daily living have been developed and much effort made in treatment of complications.

It is true to say that severe cases do so badly that some selection at the beginning is necessary. Examination of the newborn is not easy but fairly reliable criteria have been found and it is to the less-affected children that full treatment should be directed. The student will have his own opinion of the moral dilemma in these cases.

Occult spinal dysraphism

In these cases spina bifida is not obvious externally although about half will show some minor external abnormality — hairy patches, naevi, lipomatous masses, sacral pits etc.

Abnormalities of nerve roots or sometimes traction lesions on roots or spinal cord result in muscle imbalance in the legs and sphincter disturbances.

Beware the child who develops a progressive foot deformity after birth when the foot was normal at birth.

Think of the condition if treatment of a foot deformity persistently fails.

Remember that this condition is associated with sphincter imbalance and may be the cause of recurrent urinary infections.

CONGENITAL DISLOCATION OF THE HIP (0–5 years)

In this condition there is laxity, subluxation and sometimes frank dislocation of the hip at birth. It may well be that we are discussing two conditions. In the first there is joint laxity and an unfavourable intrauterine posture. In the second there is frank dysplasia of the hip. The incidence of instability at birth is about 5–10 per thousand births but only 1 per thousand persist as established dislocation.

Girls are more often affected than boys and there is a strong family and geographical association. The condition is much commoner in the countries of southern Europe.

Aetiology
1. Genetically determined joint laxity.
2. Hormonal joint laxity due to placental hormones.
3. Intrauterine posture and pressure.
4. Frank dysplasia of the hip with deficient or anteverted acetabulum and/or femoral head and intra-articular obstruction.

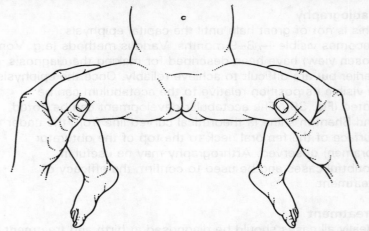

Fig. 38 Routine examination of the hips in the newborn. The examiner is abducting the hips and trying to elicit a 'click'.

Clinical features and diagnosis

1. In the neonatal period. The condition is diagnosed because it is looked for on routine examination. With the hips and knees flexed to a right angle the child's thighs are abducted (Fig. 38). A 'click' or feeling of a sudden abnormal movement alerts the examiner to the condition.
2. The established case. Many clinical features are described but the author considers only two to be reliable:
    a. Limited abduction of the hip is the most valuable sign and should be regarded as suggesting the condition until proven otherwise.
    b. If the child is walking it will have a limp. (Bilateral cases produce the well-known waddle.)

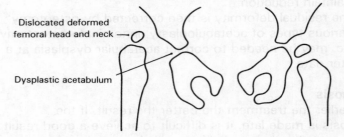

Dislocated deformed
femoral head and neck ⟶

Dysplastic acetabulum

Fig. 39 Established congenital dislocation of the hip—radiological appearance.

Radiography

This is not of great help until the capital epiphysis becomes visible — 3–9 months. Various methods (e.g. Von Rosen view) have been described for making the diagnosis earlier but are difficult to achieve reliably. Once the epiphysis is visible its position relative to the acetabulum can be noted (Fig. 39). The acetabular development can be noted, and Shenton's line (a theoretical curved line from the under surface of the femoral neck to the top of the obturator foramen) observed. Arthrography may be useful in doubtful cases and be used to confirm the efficacy of treatment.

Treatment

Ideally all cases should be diagnosed at birth and treatment started immediately. Most clinicians are content to treat the subluxatable hip with abduction in double nappies but to treat the frankly dislocated hip more vigorously on an abduction splint for approximately six weeks. The clinician should follow these cases up until he is completely satisfied that the hip is developing normally.

Treatment of the established case is much more difficult largely because diagnosis is usually delayed until the child is walking and adaptive changes have taken place. The principles are:

1. Attempts are made to reduce the hip by traction in abduction.
2. If closed reduction fails, open reduction must be performed.
3. The reduced hip is held in the acetabulum for at least six weeks with the leg in whatever position is required to maintain reduction.
4. The residual deformity is then corrected by osteotomy.
5. Various types of acetabuloplasty, innominate osteotomy etc. may be needed to correct acetabular dysplasia at a later date.

Prognosis

The earlier the treatment the better the result. If the diagnosis is made late, it is difficult to achieve a good result and osteoarthrosis later in life is a likely sequel.

THE IRRITABLE HIP (transient synovitis — under 10 years)

This term is used to describe a synovitis in the hip of young children, usually boys under 10 years of age. It is a short-lived, self-limiting inflammation of unknown aetiology.

There is pain and limitation of movements in the affected hip, particularly internal rotation. Constitutional upset is usually mild.

Treatment is by bed rest and simple traction in the early stages.

Note: The importance of this condition is that it is indistinguishable initially from such conditions as tuberculosis of the hip or Perthe's disease. Indeed acute cases may be confused with pyogenic arthritis. The clinician must follow these cases for a few months to ensure that the hip remains clinically and radiologically normal

PERTHE'S DISEASE (age 4–10 years)

This is one of the so-called osteochondritides which were previously described in this book.

It is commoner in boys and usually occurs between 4 and 10 years. The aetiology is uncertain. It is thought that there is a temporary impairment of blood supply to the capital epiphysis perhaps consequent upon an episode of synovitis with a tense effusion or swelling of the acetabular fat pad.

The condition is an avascular necrosis and the head softens, crumbles and then heals with or without deformity. Typically there is flattening or 'mushrooming' of the head. Secondary acetabular changes follow and a deformed hip may result which leads to later osteoarthrosis.

Clinical features
The condition may present like transient synovitis of the hip or more quietly with a limp and a complaint of mild pain. The child is otherwise well.

The condition is diagnosed on radiography.

Radiological changes
These follow the classic pattern of 'osteochondritis' with

sclerosis, fragmentation and healing with or without deformity. The earliest changes are an increase in joint space and slight flattening of the epiphysis (Fig. 40). Sclerosis and fragmentation follow and healing takes place over the next 2 years with or without deformity.

Certain criteria have been described which indicate the prognosis and determine treatment.

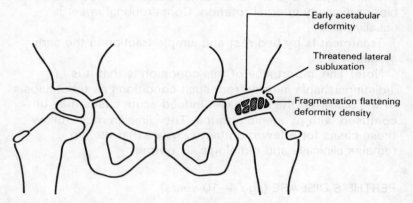

Early acetabular deformity

Threatened lateral subluxation

Fragmentation flattening deformity density

Fig. 40 The radiological appearance of Perthe's disease.

Treatment

This gives rise to much discussion. The milder cases (e.g. involving half the head) may be ignored. The more severe cases particularly those with radiological 'head at risk' signs need more energetic treatment. Younger children do well irrespective of the method of treatment.

The general principle of treatment is to obtain 'containment' of the femoral head within the acetabulum so that a well-shaped head will result. This can be achieved by abduction plasters, abduction harnesses or by varus/internal rotation osteotomy. The result of treatment of severe cases still remains unreliable. Happily in the long term even deformed hips do better than might be expected.

SLIPPED UPPER FEMORAL EPIPHYSIS (age 10–18)

This is a condition of late childhood and adolescence. The capital epiphysis slides downwards and backwards at the epiphyseal plate. This produces an adduction, external rotation and extension (loss of flexion) deformity. Ultimately the epiphyses will fuse in the deformed position.

Boys are more often affected than girls. There is an association with obesity and endocrine dysfunction. The exact cause is unknown.

Clinical features

There is a gradual onset of pain and limp. Rarely there is an acute onset associated with trauma. Note that pain may be felt in the knee.

The physical findings logically reflect the deformity. There will be pain. The leg will lie in external rotation and there will be limitation of abduction and internal rotation.

Radiographs show the epiphyseal slip. Good antero-posterior and lateral views must be obtained of both hips, for comparison. There is a risk of avascular necrosis of the capital epiphysis or cartilage necrosis. Either of these results in a severely damaged hip with pain and stiffness and early osteoarthrosis.

Treatment

This depends on the severity of the slip. Mild cases are pinned *in situ* with special pins inserted along the femoral neck. Severe cases are much more difficult. Operative reduction with shortening of the femoral neck has its advocates but it is probably safer to do a corrective osteotomy in the intertrochanteric area.

The student is asked to remember that the second hip may be at risk!

ROTATORY ABNORMALITIES OF THE LEG IN CHILDHOOD

Rotatory abnormalities of the leg in childhood usually produce intoeing. They may occur at several sites:
1.   Anteversion of the femoral neck
2.   Femoral torsion (probably not applicable in early childhood)
3.   Tibial torsion
4.   Metatarsus adductus

The clinician will be consulted because of the child's intoeing. Examination of the hip in extension will indicate the range of internal and external rotation of the hip and thus the anteversion of the femoral neck. The relative position of the patella and the foot will give a clue to tibial torsion and inspection of the underneath of the foot will show metatarsus adductus.

The angle of anteversion of the average adult femoral neck is about 15° but there is considerable individual variation. In the fetus the angle is much greater. Some children 'unwind' late and therefore have a much greater internal rotation than external rotation — hence the intoeing on walking.

About half the children with femoral neck anteversion correct spontaneously, a few do not correct at all and the remainder develop compensatory changes with external tibial torsion or everted feet. Treatment is rarely required. However, anxious parents may need much reassurance.

CONGENITAL RETROVERSION OF THE FEMORAL NECK

This is a transient condition of infancy probably due to moulding of the femoral neck by the child's posture during sleep.

The child lies with external rotation of the legs and feet and crawls with the offending foot externally rotated like a flipper. This causes great parental anxiety.

As expected the hip in extension shows limitation of internal rotation and excess external rotation.

The condition is harmless and corrects spontaneously when the child walks.

GENU VALGUM AND VARUM (knock knee and bow legs)

These conditions are common in early childhood. They are nearly always harmless and correct spontaneously.

'Genu varum' is often in fact a harmless outward curving of the tibia.

The clinician's duty is to bear in mind that certain bone diseases such as rickets or Blounts' disease may be the cause and may require treatment. Otherwise treatment is expectant with much reassurance to the parents. There is obviously a degree of severity which becomes unacceptable and surgical correction may (rarely) become necessary. This is particularly so in severe deformities in children approaching epiphyseal closure.

OSGOOD-SCHLATTER'S DISEASE

This was discussed under the heading of 'Osteochondritis'. It is an apophysitis of the tibial tuberosity, probably a fatigue or stress injury.

It usually appears in boys of 12–13 years and the child gives a good story of pain and a 'bump' well localized to the tuberosity.

X-rays show fragmentation of the tuberosity.

Treatment is in the first instance by reduction of the level of physical activity. Many cases will settle down. Acute cases may be helped by a spell in a plaster cylinder. Surgery is rarely required.

TALIPES EQUINO-VARUS (club foot) (Fig. 41)

This is a congenital deformity of the foot and ankle which has three components:
1. The ankle is in equinus (flexed).
2. The subtalar joint is inverted.
3. The forefoot is adducted.

In addition the calf is wasted and the heel small. It is often bilateral.

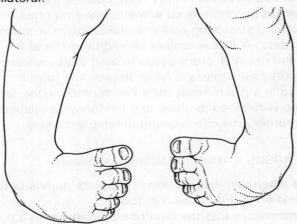

Fig. 41 Congenital talipes equino-varus (Club foot).

Aetiology

This is uncertain but the same factors as congenital dislocation of the hip must apply. (Indeed in serious multiple mesenchymal defects such as arthrogryposis multiplex congenita, both conditions commonly occur together.)

Thus we can suggest:

1. Genetically determined joint laxity.
2. Hormonal joint laxity.
3. Intrauterine position or pressure.
4. Frank dysplasia of muscles, ligaments and joints.

It is probable that club foot is caused by a failure of differentiation of specialist mesenchymal tissues or neuromuscular end plates.

Clinical features and diagnosis

The deformity is commoner in boys than girls.

The deformity is as described above.

Examination of the foot should be part of the normal postnatal check up of a newborn child.

Treatment

The principles are:

1. While it is stretchable — stretch it.
2. When it proves unstretchable — cut it.
3. If the deformity is left too long there will be bony deformity which will need bony operations.

Treatment is commenced immediately with regular manipulation, stretching and immobilization in strapping or plaster casts. A reassessment should be made at 6–12 weeks and unsatisfactory cases treated with a wide postero-medial soft tissue release. After surgery the foot is contained in a plaster cast for a few months. Long-term follow up is required as there is a tendency to relapse. Further surgery may be required in relapsed cases.

METATARSUS VARUS (metatarsus adductus)

There is often some confusion in students' minds between this condition and the true club foot.

In metatarsus varus the hindfoot is normal with a normal sized heel. The forefoot is adducted — another cause of intoeing. Many cases will correct spontaneously although passive stretching by the parents may be of assistance. In very severe cases or those with a strong dynamic component, surgery may be indicated.

TALIPES CALCANEO VALGUS

This is the opposite deformity to club foot with the foot adopting a dorsiflexed everted position. Most cases are postural but the more severe types cannot be explained by this and the aetiology is uncertain.

The condition is less 'difficult' than club foot. Passive stretching will cure many cases but the more severe ones need a period of immobilization in an overcorrected position. A few cases require surgery.

PES CAVUS (high arched foot)

This is a condition where the arch is high and weight bearing confined to the metatarsal heads and the heel (Fig. 42). Many cases have claw toes as well which again increases the load on the metatarsal heads.

About half the cases can be shown to have a neurological basis, albeit minor. Some cases are familial.

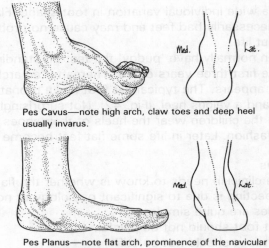

Pes Cavus—note high arch, claw toes and deep heel usually invarus.

Pes Planus—note flat arch, prominence of the navicular tuberosity and heel in valgus

Fig. 42 Pes Cavus and Pes Planus.

Clinical features

The condition becomes evident in childhood and adolescence. The problems are those of overload on the metatarsal heads with pain. Painful callosities may develop under the metatarsal heads, on the toes and even on the dorsum of the foot where shoes cause pressure.

The spine should be checked for evidence of spinal dysraphism and a neurological examination performed.

Treatment

Mild cases require no treatment or can be managed with chiropody, pressure relieving insoles etc.

In severe cases surgery may be required. If the heel is straight it is worthwhile doing a soft tissue (Steindler) release on the sole of the foot. If the heel is in varus a corrective osteotomy of the calcaneum may improve foot shape. If claw toes are the problem, fusion of the interphalangeal joints is required so that the long flexors may help to relieve weight on the metatarsal heads, and pressure on the dorsal surface of the proximal interphalangeal joints relieved.

PES PLANUS (flat foot)

There is a wide individual variation in foot shape. Flat feet are not necessarily bad feet and may cause no problems throughout life.

Children normally have 'pudgy' flat feet on standing during the first three years of life. Thereafter an arch gradually appears. The typical flat foot has a pronated forefoot and a valgus heel. (Fig. 42). Not surprisingly therefore the children wear the heels of their shoes over in 'valgus' fashion. Later in life some flat feet become painful.

Diagnosis

What the clinician needs to know is whether the flat foot he is inspecting is due to significant pathology or not.

The rules are quite simple:
1.   A flat foot should not be painful.
2.   A flat foot should not be stiff.
3.   The arch should restore when the child stands on tiptoe.

If any of these abnormal features are present the clinician

should consider the possibility of congenital anomaly or inflammatory arthritis.

Diagnosis

Mild flat foot requires no treatment. If the heel is in marked valgus or shoe distortion severe, then the use of a heel-cup insole will be of value. Longitudinal arch supports are advocated by some. It is doubtful whether the exercises practised in the past have any value. Severe persisting flat foot may require surgery — usually directed at stabilizing the subtalar joint to straighten the heel.

'OSTEOCHONDRITIS' OF THE NAVICULAR BONE (Kohler's disease)

This has been dealt with elsewhere. The student is asked to remember that this condition may be a cause of foot pain in young children.

'OSTEOCHONDRITIS' OF THE SECOND METATARSAL HEAD (Freiberg's disease)

This curious condition of adolescent girls causes pain well localized to the joint concerned and radiographs confirm the diagnosis.

TOE DEFORMITIES

These are common in childhood but are rarely a problem.
Extra digits may occur.
'Curly' toes or under-riding toes cause parental anxiety, but are usually self correcting.
Digitus Quintus Varus is a condition in which the little toe over-rides the 4th toe. It usually requires surgical correction. Hammer toe is a condition caused by a fixed flexion deformity of the proximal interphalangeal joint with overlying callosity. Surgical fusion cures the condition.

CEREBRAL PALSY (spastic child)

This name is given to a group of syndromes arising as a result of brain damage during development, birth or early infancy. The commonest cause is an episode of anoxia but birth trauma and head injury after birth may occur.

The name 'spastic' is a poor one, as it describes the peripheral and mainly motor effect of a disease which has equally important central effects.

Central effects — Mental deficiency.
                — Late development
                — Poor balance
                — Fits
                — Visual defects
                — Poor speech

Peripheral effects — Spasticity
                  — Rigidity
                  — Athetosis
                  — Ataxia
                  — Atonia (rare type)
                  — Exclusion of an extremity from the 'body image'.

Diagnosis

The early diagnosis is often difficult. A late case will present with evident upper motor neurone signs and some of the above features.

Early evidence:
1. History of abnormal pregnancy, prematurity, abnormal delivery or crisis in early life.
2. Delayed development.
3. Abnormal reflex patterns.
4. Tight adductor muscles of the hips—often found accidentally while checking the hips routinely.
5. Gait abnormalities.

Management

The student should understand that the management of cerebral palsy is multidisciplinary involving:
Paediatric neurologist
Paediatric physiotherapist
Speech therapist
Educational psychologist
Audiologist
Social worker
The parents

The role of the orthopaedic surgeon is a modest one. He or she joins the team to select such cases as may benefit from surgery and then to carry out that surgery. The student is reminded that these children may need continuous care and help from the team until adulthood. Less than 10% of all cases require surgery.

Generally the team will choose a child without severe mental handicap, who seems motivated, has adequate balance and who does not suffer from uncontrolled abnormal movements. The selection of patients and of the operations proposed requires considerable experience of the condition and the details are not within the scope of this small book.

OTHER NEUROLOGICAL DISORDERS PRESENTING IN CHILDHOOD

1. Anterior poliomyelitis. Lower motor neurone paralysis affecting all ages and associated with a febrile illness and signs of cerebral or meningeal irritation caused by poliovirus.
2. Peripheral neuritis (Guillain-Barre syndrome). May be viral but chemical poisoning also occurs. Tends to be symmetrical and there are CSF changes.
3. Birth injuries. Usually upper limb and associated with difficult deliveries. These are brachial plexus injuries.
   a. Upper type (Erbs palsy) — shoulder movement and biceps affected.
   b. Lower type (Klumpke's palsy) — forearm and hand affected.
4. Congenital absence of pain. Suspect this when bizarre multiple fractures or neuropathic joints occur in children.
5. Peroneal muscular atrophy. Peripheral motor nerves and later spinal cord affected. Family history. Progressive foot deformities occur from age of 5 years.

MUSCULAR DYSTROPHY

The child is born normal.
   Usually male child 5–10 years affected.
   Presents with tiredness, weakness, odd gait and sometimes pseudo-hypertrophy of calves.

Investigations include muscle biopsy, electromyography, serum aldolase and creatinine kinase estimation.

The disease is often sex linked and transmitted to boys via the mother. Investigation and handling of parents may require great care.

There is no specific treatment but the affected children may need bracing, splinting, calipers etc. Surgical correction of deformity may aid the orthotist.

DWARFISM

A simplified classification of dwarfism follows:
1. Proportional dwarfism. Mucopolysaccharidoses e.g. Hunter–Hurler disease. Metabolic disorders, e.g. Rickets.
2. Short limb dwarfism. Achondroplasia. Diastrophic dwarfism. Osteogenesis imperfecta.
3. Short trunk dwarfism. Spondylo-epiphyseal dysplasia. Severe Scheurmann's Disease. Metatropic dwarfism in teenage.
4. Other endocrine disorders. Cretinism (hypothyroidism). Hypopituitarism (occasionally).

GENERALIZED DISORDERS OF THE SKELETON

This section tends to intimidate students with multiple eponyms and lists of similar conditions with slight differences. It is not necessary for the undergraduate student to know the details of these conditions. Remember that they may be associated with dwarfism, growth abnormalities, epiphyseal irregularity, widespread bone and joint disease and skeletal deformity.

A brief classification is given and a few lines offered concerning the clinically more important conditions.

1. Diseases of the epiphysis

Diastrophic dwarfism is chosen for mention here in that it resembles achondroplasia clinically but is transmitted by an autosomal gene — the risk to siblings is high.

2. Disease of the growth plate

Achondroplasia is the commonest cause of dwarfism. These dwarfs are well known to all children as the typical circus dwarfs:
   a. Large head with small face and saddle nose.
   b. Relatively large trunk.

   c.   Short limbs.
   d.   Deep lumbar lordosis and small pelvis.
   e.   Usually mutant gene responsible.

Dyschondroplasia is a condition in which there is a failure of orderly ossification in the growth plate resulting in multiple chondromas.

3   Diseases of the metaphysis

Diaphyseal Aclasis—think of this condition in patients who have multiple osteochondromata.

4   Diseases of the diaphysis

Osteogenesis Imperfecta is a familial disease in which there is a failure to form normal bone matrix cf. adult osteoporosis. Severity varies from stillbirth, bedridden dwarfs with multiple fractures and unclosed skull sutures to relatively normal individuals who suffer repeated fractures. The long bones are narrow, porotic and thin in the cortex. Deformity is common. The sclera are often blue and hypotonia often associated. Prophylactic intramedullary nailing may benefit some of these cases.

CAUSES OF LIMP IN CHILDHOOD

1. Trauma — many injuries in children go unnoticed. Greenstick fractures are often only recognized on X-ray.
2. Pain of other cause. This could be from any cause from standing on a drawing pin to the onset of a bone tumour.
3. Instability at the hip. This gives the typical instability gait when the centre of gravity is thrown over the diseased hip. The student is asked to think of power, fulcrum and levers. Failure of any these produces the limp, hence:
   Hip joint disease or subluxation.
   Muscle weakness.
   Coxa vara.
4. Muscle weakness, e.g. muscular dystrophy.
5. Neurological disorder. Lower motor neurone, e.g. weak glutei or drop foot. Upper motor neurone, e.g. cerebral palsy.
6. Inequality of leg length.
7. Hysteria.

CAUSES OF MULTIPLE PERIOSTITIS

Multiple trauma (includes non-accidental injury)
Multiple osteomyelitis
Scurvy
Syphilis
Infantile cortical hyperostosis (mandible involved as well)

NON-ACCIDENTAL INJURY (battered baby syndrome)

This is a delicate subject in which the clinician has to balance the sensitivities of the parents concerned against the risk to the child. Remember that one good tumble downstairs could produce several injuries.

What the clinician needs to observe is whether there is evidence of several injuries which have obviously occurred at different times.

The typical 'Orthopaedic' presentation is that of repeated visits for fracture and X-rays showing old healed fractures, periostitis and metaphyseal chip fractures.

If these features are present the child should be regarded as at serious risk, particularly from head injury.

The clinician should consult with a specialist paediatrician after which the condition is dealt with on a multidisciplinary basis with reports from health visitors, school teachers, social workers etc.

WHAT IS THE CAUSE OF . . . ?

If the student is asked, 'What is the cause of this condition' and finds himself or herself intellectually destitute, a reasonable answer can usually be found under the following headings. These should be learnt.

1. Congenital
2. Traumatic
3. Inflammatory — Acute (indicates infection)
   — Chronic
4. Neoplastic — Primary
   — Secondary
5. Degenerative
6. Vascular
7. Neurological
8. Endocrine

9. Metabolic
10. System diseases (collagen diseases)
11. Mechanical
12. Calculi (do not usually fit elsewhere in the classification)
13. Iatrogenic

Backache (including 'back—buttock—leg pain)

Backache is an extremely common complaint and accounts for over one million referrals to general practitioners each year. The majority of these concern the lumbar spine. In orthopaedic outpatients, low back pain is responsible for about 20–25% of referrals.

EXAMINATION OF THE SPINE

This has been discussed elsewhere (see p. 114).

CAUSES OF BACKACHE

Congenital:	Spondylolysis
	Spondylolisthesis
	Scoliosis or kyphoscoliosis
	Spina bifida
	Hemivertebra
Traumatic:	Vertebral fracture and fracture-dislocation
	Muscle or ligament tears
	Joint strain
	Intervertebral disc prolapse
Inflammatory:	Infection — Discitis
	— Osteomyelitis
	Ankylosing spondylitis
	Other rheumatological disorders
Degenerative:	Osteoarthrosis — disc narrowing
	— posterior intervetebral joint arthritis
	— spinal stenosis
Metabolic:	Osteoporosis
	Osteomalacia
	Paget's disease (unknown aetiology)

Neoplastic: Metastatic deposits in bone
                 Primary tumours of bone or neural
                 tissues
Visceral: Retroperitoneal tumours, e.g carcinoma
                 of body of pancreas.
Gynaecological: Pelvic inflammatory disease
                 Endometriosis
Vascular: Aortic aneurysm
                 Dissecting aneurysm
                 High claudication, i.e. aorto-iliac occlusion
                 Note that the claudication may give rise
                 to back—buttock—leg pain!
Mechanical: Poor posture is often associated with
                 mild backache.
Psychogenic: Musculoskeletal pain is probably the
                 commonest presentation of
                 psychosomatic disorder and much of this
                 is back pain. Unfortunately it is common
                 to find organic disease accompanied by a
                 psychological overlay which hinders
                 diagnosis and impairs treatment.

DIAGNOSIS OF LOW BACK PAIN

The student is encouraged to think of back—buttock—leg
pain as a symptom complex. The history may leave the
clinician in doubt as to which structure is actually involved
but systematic examination will identify this. Some other
useful points are:

1. Pain on flexion tends to originate in disc pathology.
2. Pain on extension tends to originate in facet joint
    pathology.
3. Pain on movement sounds 'orthopaedic'.
4. Continuous pain suggests neoplasia, erosion of bone or
    psychogenic disease.
5. Tension signs indicate dural or nerve root irritation.
6. True nerve root pain is usually accurately described.
7. Referred pain is less well described.
8. Always ask about trauma.
9. Always ask about other joint involvement.
10. Remember the five carcinomata which metastasize to
    bone.
11. Beware the stiff painful back in children.

COMMON CONDITIONS OF THE SPINE

Infection, neoplasia and the polyarthritides have been discussed elsewhere.

Osteoarthrosis in the spine

Disc degeneration causes disc narrowing. This mechanical alteration predisposes the posterior intervertebral joints to osteoarthrosis. This gives rise to:

1. Pain in facet joints sometimes referred to buttock or thigh.
2. Osteophytes may encroach on intervertebral foramina and cause root irritation.
3. Osteoarthritic facet joints may subluxate and allow spondylolisthesis.
4. Osteophyte encroachment or a narrow spinal canal may cause spinal stenosis.

Radiography shows disc narrowing and osteophyte formation.

Treatment

The majority of cases are managed conservatively by:

Simple analgesics

Non-steroidal anti-inflammatory drugs

Physiotherapy — heat or shortwave diathermy

— exercises

— mobilization and manipulation

Corset

A good rule of thumb is that the patient who is better at rest will do well with a back support or corset and the patient who is better up and about will do well with physiotherapy. Attention to weight, limitation of heavy activities and instruction in back care, sleeping posture etc. are important adjuncts to more active therapy. Severe intractable pain may occasionally require surgical fusion with or without decompression but careful assessment of the case is essential. The history should be reviewed, the clinical condition and special investigations re-examined and the previous treatment evaluated. A psychological assessment may be of help. Certain poor prognosis patients may be thus excluded.

If surgery is contemplated it should only be after full discussion with the patient to ensure that the expectations of the patient match those of the surgeon and that the patient understands what is involved.

Osteochondritis (Scheurmann's disease)
This is one of the osteochondritides discussed elsewhere. However, there are some important points to mention.

It is the cause of adolescent round back. A gradual curve or kyphosis occurs. Some backache, not usually severe, may be associated. Radiating pain is rare. The patients are often tall, slim, 'droopy' with tight hamstrings.

X-rays show wedging of vertebrae and irregularity of the vertebral endplates.

Treatment
The majority of cases are mild, self limiting and require no treatment. Postural exercises may help to improve the appearance. A minority of the more severe cases need bracing in a spinal brace or even spinal fusion.

Spondylolysis and Spondylolisthesis
Spondylolysis is a defect in the neural arch usually in the pars interarticularis of the 4th or 5th lumbar vertebra. The gap may be congenital or traumatic in origin. It fills with fibrous tissue and is therefore unable to offer the same resistance to antero-posterior shearing stresses as healthy vertebrae. If as a consequence of this the upper of the vertebrae begins to shift forward on the lower we have a spondylolisthesis (Fig. 43).

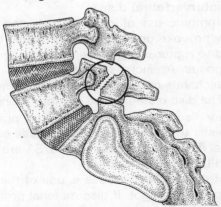

Fig. 43 Spondylolisthesis with the area of mechanical failure encircled.

There are three main groups:
1. Spondylolysis (defect in neural arch)
    — Congenital
    — Traumatic
    — acute
    — Chronic
2. Congenital deficiency of facet joints
3. Degenerative—osteoarthritic joints become so damaged that forward slip can occur.

Clinical features of spondylolisthesis
The patient usually presents with chronic backache worse on standing. Occasionally there may be sciatica and symptoms or signs of nerve root irritation or compression.

Spondylolisthesis is one of the causes of spinal stenosis.
    The condition is diagnosed by radiography. Oblique films may be needed to demonstrate a defect in the pars interarticularis.

Treatment
In general bad 'slips' of congenital origin in young people have a much worse prognosis than mild slips of degenerative origin in older people. Mild cases may require only analgesics and a lumbosacral corset. Severe symptoms or a demonstrable severe or progressive 'slip' may necessitate surgery by decompression and fusion of the spine at the level of the 'slip'.

Prolapsed intervertebral disc
This is a common cause of low back pain and sciatica. Trauma may provoke onset but it is probable that the disc is predisposed to rupture by degenerative changes in the nucleus pulposus. An increase of short-chain mucopolysaccharide molecules causes an osmotic attraction. The disc distends and is more prone to rupture.
    Almost any disc may be involved but for practical purposes this is to be regarded as a disease of the lower lumbar spine. The discs between L4/5/S1 are most affected and L3/4 rather less so.
    Rupture of the annulus fibrosus is one of the causes of acute back pain (lumbago). If disc material prolapses through the rent in the annulus it may act as an extradural mass

and irritate dura and nerve root — thus causing sciatica and other radicular symptoms and signs. The shape and size of the patients spinal canal also influences the presentation of the disease.

Clinical features
There is usually a history of strain or mild injury, e.g. bending or lifting. The patient is aware of 'something happening in my back'. Backache follows. Onset may be acute or gradual. Sciatica and radicular symptoms often appear later. Pain is worse on bending, lifting, coughing and sneezing. Note that urinary symptoms herald disaster and should not be ignored.

Examination reveals a stiffly held back often with a total (or sciatic) scoliosis tilting to one side (Fig. 44) The lumbar spine is often flattened and muscle spasm is evident. Movements are cautious and painful, particularly flexion. There may be local tenderness over the interspinous ligament at the affected level.

The straight leg raising test is usually positive.

The student should look for patterns of neurological deficit rather than examining everything.

L3/4 prolapse — quadriceps weakness, depressed or absent knee jerk, sensory signs unreliable.

L4/5 prolapse — no reflex involved
weakness of extensor hallucis longus, foot dorsiflexors and evertors hypoaesthesia on lateral side of calf and medial side of foot

L5/S1 prolapse — depressed or absent ankle jerk hypoaesthesia on lateral side of foot.

Radiography may be of little help in acute cases. It excludes the unexpected. It may confirm the scoliosis and the loss of lumbar lordosis. In chronic cases disc narrowing may be visible. Computerized axial tomography (and in the future, nuclear magnetic resonance) may be of help in difficult cases.

Myelography or radiculography is an invasive procedure (injecting contrast media into the theca) and should only be performed where there is serious doubt about the diagnosis or where surgery is a strong possibility.

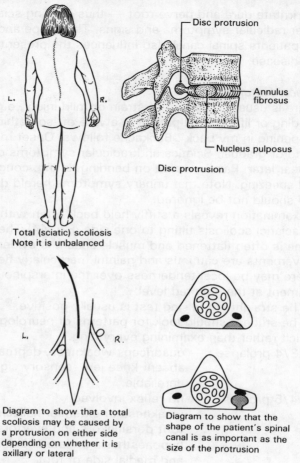

Total (sciatic) scoliosis
Note it is unbalanced

Diagram to show that a total scoliosis may be caused by a protrusion on either side depending on whether it is axillary or lateral

Diagram to show that the shape of the patient's spinal canal is as important as the size of the protrusion

Fig. 44 Prolapsed intervertebral disc.

Treatment

The majority of cases will get better with analgesics, bed rest with or without traction. Severe cases need to be hospitalized. Mild cases may need only a corset or other back support.

It is reasonable for a general practitioner to put a patient with acute low back pain to bed for a week or ten days. BUT he must have examined the patient thoroughly to exclude the unexpected and he should not ignore a neurological deficit or any bladder symptoms. A patient who is not better in ten days should be referred to hospital.

The reason that patients get better spontaneously is that the herniated material shrinks and the rent heals.

Surgery to remove the prolapse is indicated in two circumstances and should be preceded by radiculography:

1. Severe pain unrelieved by adequate conservative treatment.
2. Severe neurological disturbance. Note that cauda equina compression threatening bladder function should be regarded as a surgical emergency.

Spinal stenosis

Spinal stenosis is a self-descriptive name. The spinal canal is narrowed. Usually this is a combination of a narrow canal and intruding osteophytes from osteoarthritic facet joints or distortion of the canal such as occurs in spondylolisthesis. The most important clinical feature is that of spinal claudication, i.e. pain in back, buttocks, and legs on exercise. This is due to dural or nerve root irritation. It may resemble high vascular claudication. There may be patchy sensory disturbances but usually not much else on examination. A typical feature is that the pain is eased by rest in flexed position and it is said that exercise with the spine flexed, e.g. cycling does not induce the symptoms found when exercise is taken erect.

Diagnosis and treatment

Where the condition is suspected it must be confirmed with myelography, computerized axial tomography or even ultrasound measurement. A proven case is treated by spinal decompression. Mild or doubtful cases are best treated conservatively.

Backache and the sacro-iliac joint

Any inflammation involving a sacro-iliac joint will present as backache. Acute and chronic infections do occur rarely but the most important example of this is the sacro-iliitis of ankylosing spondylitis (and other sero-negative polyarthritides). The joint is often involved in trauma of the pelvis and may be painful after pregnancy or labour.

'Sacro-iliac strain' is a dubious entity but probably does exist occasionally. The majority of cases are probably of referred pain from the lumbar spine. However, the diagnosis is often made by those skilled in manipulative medicine who claim considerable success resulting from 'manipulation' of the joints.

Coccydynia

This name refers to any condition causing pain in the region of the coccyx. The condition is vexacious to both the patient and the orthopaedic surgeon.

Examination must include the lumbar spine, the sacro-iliac joints and pelvic examination. A rectal examination is mandatory to exclude intrapelvic or rectal pathology and also to demonstrate whether moving the coccyx itself reproduces the pain.

The majority of cases are due to trauma. Typically the patient has a fall in the sitting position thus straining the sacro-coccygeal joint or contusing the coccyx and lower sacrum. The patient has pain on sitting but not on standing or lying. Local tenderness and pain on moving the coccyx suggest a traumatic origin. Radiographs are usually negative but occasionally a fracture of the lower sacrum may be found.

Unfortunately some patients have no history of injury. In these cases the surgeon must exclude other causes, e.g. tumours of sacrum or coccyx, pelvic disease, pain referred from lumbar spine, local infections or even psychogenic disorders.

Treatment of the traumatic type is expectant. Reassurance and analgesics are given. Other treatments such as shortwave diathermy or local hydrocortisone injections are sometimes recommended but unreliable. In very exceptional cases, excision of the coccyx may be a last resort.

Neck–shoulder–arm pain and miscellaneous conditions of the upper limb

The student is encouraged to think of neck–shoulder–arm pain as an entity because it is such a common symptom complex in general practice and orthopaedic practice. Thinking in this way ensures that all the relevant common conditions are considered.

CERVICAL SPONDYLOSIS

Degenerative disease of the cervical spine occurs early and radiological changes may be found in young adults. The disease affects the intervertebral discs with narrowing and osteophyte formation, and the posterior intervertebral joints where osteoarthrosis develops. Loss of movement, particularly lateral flexion is usual in middle-aged people but there are often no symptoms, i.e. radiological changes correlate poorly with symptoms. Mild symptoms such as slight pain, creaking and clicking are common but as with osteoarthritic joints elsewhere acute exacerbations occur. It is usually such an exacerbation which makes the patient seek advice.

The acute attack of cervical spondylosis usually occurs spontaneously with pain and stiffness in the neck and often across one shoulder. Pain is often referred across the shoulder and vaguely distributed down the upper arm. True radicular pain may be provoked by intrusion of a swollen posterior intervertebral joint into an exit foramen already narrowed by osteophytes (Fig. 45). The nerve root is irritated. This radicular pain extends from the base of the neck, across the shoulder and down the arm often to the hand. It may be associated with pain and paraesthesia in one or more digits. Muscle weakness or 'objective' hypoaesthesia are less common. The pain is sometimes referred up to the occipital region.

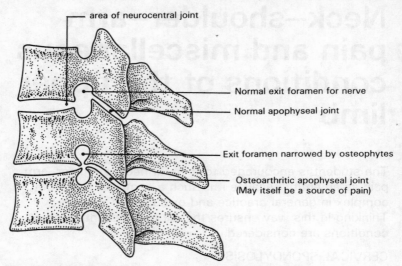

Fig. 45 Cervical spondylosis—diagram to illustrate sources of pain in neck–shoulder–arm.

Examination should include the cervical spine, the neck and the supraclavicular triangles, the shoulders, the axillae, the great nerve trunks in the affected arm, reflexes, power and sensation. Remember that the middle finger represents the C7 root and everything else is distributed evenly on each side. Pain and stiffness is immediately apparent and the patient often holds the neck in a slightly odd or flexed position.

True prolapse of intervertebral discs into the cervical canal is probably rare but longstanding changes may be associated with a myelopathy giving rise to upper motor neurone signs in the legs. True disc prolapse is only likely to be diagnosed when objective neurological signs are impressive and then it is difficult to distinguish from other lesions such as spinal cord or extradural tumours.

Special investigations
Radiography will show degenerative changes and oblique films may show exit foramen narrowing. Myelography is rarely indicated. In the future computerized axial tomography or nuclear majnetic resonance may become the investigations of choice.

Treatment
Treatment of the acute attack of pain is usually by analgesics, non-steroidal anti-inflammatory drugs and support (temporary collar). Physiotherapy often helps. Traction is of value but manipulations may be dangerous. In recalcitrant cases the wearing of a purpose made cervical collar for some weeks may be necessary. Surgery is rarely indicated.

CERVICAL RIB

Cervical ribs are congenital abnormalities of the 7th cervical vertebra wherein the transverse process or an attached costal process may extend as a bony projection or fibrous band down towards the first rib. Many cases of pain and neurological symptoms in the arm formerly attributed to cervical rib probably arise in cervical spondylosis. However, cervical rib may occasionally be responsible for pain, paraesthesiae and numbness in the upper limb.

More commonly, however, cervical ribs (which are usually symptomless) give rise to vascular problems associated with subclavian artery stenosis, post-stenotic dilatation and the release of small mural emboli down the brachial artery. This is one cause of Raynaud's phenomenon. In such cases abnormal pulsation, arterial bruits or absent or reduced wrist pulses may be found.

Palpation of the supraclavicular triangles has already been recommended in cases of neck pain. Some cervical ribs are palpable. The remainder will be visible on the antero-posterior film of the neck or on a standard chest X-ray.

Treatment
In the few cases with proven neurological deficit or vascular symptoms the cervical rib may need to be excised.

There are other presumed congenital abnormalities (such as scalenus anterior syndrome) in the same region which may simulate cervical rib syndrome.

NEURALGIC AMYOTROPHY AND OTHER LOCALIZED NEURITIDES

A rare cause of acute neck–shoulder–arm pain is the localized neuritis of neuralgic amyotrophy. These neuritides are thought to be viral in origin and curiously affect mainly the muscles of the shoulder and shoulder girdle.

Think of the condition when there is a sudden onset of severe neck—shoulder—arm pain without trauma. Typically the painful period lasts for a few days after which muscle paralysis in the deltoid (less often other scapular muscles, e.g. the winged scapula of serratus anterior palsy) are affected. The biceps jerk may be depressed. Electromyography may aid diagnosis.

In most cases the paralysis recovers to a greater or lesser extent. Physiotherapy may assist recovery.

CAPSULITIS OF THE SHOULDER, FROZEN SHOULDER AND PAINFUL ARC SYNDROME

The shoulder capsule is very elastic permitting a wide range of movement. The glenoid is small and shallow and the stability of the shoulder is 'dynamic' depending on several tendons which are intimately associated with the capsule. Also in close proximity are several bursae, notably the subacromial bursa — hence any trauma or inflammation may effect one or more movements of the shoulder with pain or stiffness.

In some patients during middle life an ill-understood low-grade inflammation of part or most of the shoulder capsule occurs. The histology shows low-grade non-specific inflammatory changes. The disease results in pain and loss of elasticity of the capsule. If the area involved includes a bursa or tendon then we may see a symptom complex characterized by pain during a specific arc of movement. Hence the presentation of this disease depends not only on the pathology but also the localization of that pathology. We call this inflammation 'capsulitis'. The aetiology is unknown but presumably degenerative disease plays a part. Interestingly the same patients may develop similar problems elsewhere over a period of a few years.

1. If a large part of the capsule is involved we see a 'Frozen Shoulder'. There is pain lasting days or weeks followed by stiffness lasting months. Pain decreases as stiffness increases. The natural history runs over a period of 18—24 months after which some improvement occurs spontaneously.

2. If the area of the subacromial bursa is involved we see a painful arc syndrome affecting mid abduction. The patient can initiate abduction but as the greater tuberosity passes under the acromion, pain and sometimes inhibition of abduction occurs (Fig. 46).

3. If the area of the supraspinatus tendon is involved we see a painful arc in the early part of abduction, i.e. when the supraspinatus tendon is most involved and again when the inflamed area passes under the acromion.

4. If the long head of biceps is involved there may be a painful inhibition of flexion/abduction particularly if the forearm is held supinated.

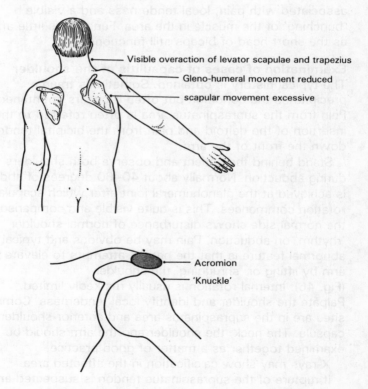

Fig. 46 *Above:* The classic 'shrug' of the patient trying to abduct a painful shoulder. *Below:* Illustration to show how the 'knuckle' of the greater tuberosity of the humerus squeezes the capsule or subacromial bursa against the acromion in mid abduction—hence possible painful arc syndrome.

Further degenerative changes may lead to rupture

Rupture of the supraspinatus tendon
Although this tendon may be ruptured by trauma it is probable
that the majority of cases occur in a tendon already degenerate.
The diagnosis is made by obtaining a history of trauma with
local tenderness and inability to initiate abduction. Note that the
deltoid can sustain abduction but not initiate it. X-rays
sometimes show calcification in the tendon.

Rupture of the long head of biceps tendon
Similarly to the above this rupture probably occurs in a
previously diseased tendon. A history of trauma is
associated with pain, local tenderness and a visible
'bunching' of the muscle in the area. Function is little affected
as the short head of biceps still functions.

Examination of cases of capsulitis of the shoulder
The typical history is obtained. Sometimes trauma
precipitates the condition but often it occurs spontaneously.
Pain from the supraspinatus area is often referred to the
insertion of the deltoid and pain from the bicipital tendon
down the front of the arm.

Stand behind the patient and observe both shoulders
during abduction. Normally about 40–60 degrees of abduction
is achieved at the glenohumeral joint after which scapular
rotation commences. This is quite visible and comparison with
the normal side shows disturbance of normal shoulder
'rhythm' on abduction. Pain may be obvious and typical
abnormal feature is that the patient attempts to elevate the
arm by lifting or 'shrugging' the shoulder
(Fig. 46). Internal rotation is usually markedly limited.
Palpate the shoulder and identify local tenderness. Common
sites are in the supraspinatus area and anterior shoulder
capsule. The neck, the shoulder and the arm should be
examined together as a matter of good practice.

X-rays may show calcification in the affected area.

If rupture of the supraspinatus tendon is suspected an
arthrogram may demonstrate the lesion.

Treatment of capsulitis of the shoulder
Mild cases may need only mild analgesics or a course of
non-steroidal anti-inflammatory drugs.

It is probable that physiotherapy has little benefit in these cases except as an adjunct to other therapy, i.e. to restore movement.

Injection of the affected area with hydrocortisone and local anaesthetic often benefits these cases, and confers the benefit of aiding diagnosis. If the symptoms are relieved by the local anaesthetic the diagnosis is confirmed.

A totally frozen shoulder may be helped by manipulation under anaesthesia if hydrocortisone is injected at the same time. Complete ruptures of the supraspinatus tendon may need repair.

OSTEOARTHRITIS OF THE ACROMIOCLAVICULAR JOINT

This condition may mimic capsulitis in that there may be pain on abduction. However, tenderness can usually be localized to the joint itself.

MISCELLANEOUS CONDITIONS OF THE UPPER LIMB

Recurrent dislocation of the shoulder

Following a known traumatic dislocation of the shoulder further episodes of dislocation occur often with trivial trauma or strain.

The condition is usually due to tearing of the capsule and glenoid labrum off the glenoid margin thus leaving a permanent defect or pouch into which anterior dislocation of the humeral head may occur recurrently.

The condition is diagnosed by the story but before proceeding to treatment at least one of the episodes of dislocation should be observed and recorded radiologically.

Treatment is surgical. There are several operations in common use. The principle of all is to close the defect and to tighten the anterior capsule.

Referred pain to the shoulder

Remember that occasionally pain may arise in the shoulder from lesions of the neck, cervical nerve roots, apex of the lung and irritation of the diaphragmatic pleura or peritoneum.

Tennis elbow (lateral epicondylitis)

This is a condition in which there is a chronic inflammation of the origin of the extensor muscles of the forearm at the lateral epicondyle.

It is usually due to repeated stress, e.g. tennis playing but some cases have no obvious explanation.

The pain is well localized and usually felt on gripping strongly. The pain may radiate down the back of the forearm. Flexing and pronating the wrist and extending the elbow may exacerbate the pain. Tenderness is precisely localized to the extensor origin on the epicondyle.

Treatment

Hydrocortisone and local anaesthetic injected into the tender area usually cures the condition after one or more treatments. Surgery is rarely indicated.

Golfer's elbow (medial epicondylitis)

This is less common but similar condition affecting the medial epicondyle. Treatment is along the same lines but beware the close proximity of the ulnar nerve.

Ulnar neuritis

The ulnar nerve is vulnerable to pressure or chronic friction as it lies in the ulnar groove behind the medial epicondyle. Forearm pain and numbness or paraesthesiae in the ulnar two digits of the hand are the usual symptoms. In severe cases objective hypoaesthesia and wasting or weakness of the intrinsic muscles of the hand may be detected. Sometimes the classic 'ulnar claw hand' may be observed. Here there is inability of the patient actively to extend the interphalangeal joints of the ulnar side digits.

Diagnosis can be confirmed by electrodiagnostic studies. Treatment is by transposition of the ulnar nerve to a new bed anterior to the medial epicondyle.

Tenosynovitis of the forearm

This is a frictional tenosynovitis usually in the distal part of the extensor compartment. It is caused by vigorous activity, e.g. rowing.

Pain, tenderness and crepitus are the usual feature's.

Treatment is by rest, by support and by non-steroidal anti-inflammatory drugs.

Osteoarthrosis of the wrist and hand

Osteoarthrosis of the wrist is not common and is usually secondary to previous disease, e.g. non-union of a fracture of the scaphoid bone.

However, certain sites are typical of the osteoarthrosis of postmenopausal women. The trapezio-metacarpal joints and the distal interphalangeal joints are typically so affected.

Kienbock's disease of the lunate

This is one of the 'osteochondritides' described elsewhere in the book. Think of this condition in cases of persisting wrist pain in young adults and exclude it radiologically.

Flexor tenosynovitis

The flexor tendons and their synovial sheaths may be affected in chronic inflammatory conditions such as rheumatoid arthritis and tuberculosis. When longstanding inflammation is present, considerable swelling may occur leading to the diagnosis of 'Compound palmar ganglion'.

De Quervain's tenovaginitis

This is an inflammatory condition usually of uncertain origin affecting the fibrous sheath of tendons of abductor pollicis longus and extensor pollicis brevis as they cross the radial styloid.

The condition may be acute or chronic. If chronic the lesion may produce a palpable lump.

Pain and tenderness are well localized and the pain may be provoked by passive ulnar deviation of the whole hand and thumb together.

Treatment is by division of the sheath but very acute cases may respond to local steroid injection.

Carpal tunnel syndrome

This is a condition in which the median nerve is compressed in the carpal tunnel. Most cases occur due to non-specific thickening of the transverse carpal ligament in middle age. However, any condition predisposing to fluid retention or tissue thickening in the tunnel may cause the symptoms. Hence we find it in rheumatoid arthritis, pregnancy, use of contraceptive hormones, myxoedema etc. Distortion of the tunnel by fracture may also cause the condition.

The typical patient is a middle-aged woman. She complains of clumsiness, numbness and paraesthesiae in the hand (usually the patient herself does not volunteer that the little finger is unaffected) and pain up the arm. The symptoms are typically worse at night. Objective findings are usually not present but if they are will consist of hypoaesthesia in the distribution of the median nerve and weakness and wasting of the muscles of the thenar eminence.

Electrodiagnostic studies usually confirm the diagnosis but it is advisable for the student to remember that similar symptoms may arise from disease in the neck, the axilla, or nerve trunks of the arm.

Carpal tunnel syndrome may be cured by surgical decompression of the tunnel, dividing the transverse carpal ligament.

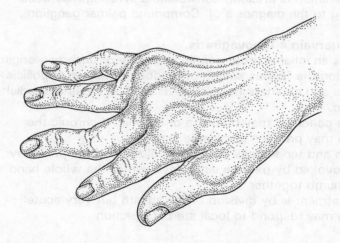

Fig. 47 Diagram to show the feature of rheumatoid arthritis of the hand. Note the synovial swelling and subluxation of the metacarpo-phalangeal joints, ulnar deviation at wrist and fingers. A Boutonniere deformity is demonstrated at the little finger and swan-neck deformity at the middle finger.

Rheumatoid arthritis of the wrist and hand

Although this disease has been discussed elsewhere, it is valuable to repeat that the disease often commences in the hand and when advanced is often most noticeable in the hand and wrist:

1. Metacarpophalangeal joints of the thumb and fingers with swelling, subluxation and the classic ulnar drift of the fingers (Fig. 47).
2. Proximal interphalangeal joints of the fingers.
3. The wrist joint, particularly involving the inferior radioulnar joint.
4. The flexor tendons — tenosynovitis, triggering and attrition ruptures.
5. The intrinsic muscles with contracture and classic swan neck deformity.
6. Masses of rheumatoid synovium may make 'lumps' on the extensor surfaces.

Note that the distal interphalangeal joints are not usually affected, If they are then the presence of another type of polyarthritis should be suspected.

7. Two typical deformities of the fingers deserve special mention (see Fig. 47).
   a. Swan neck deformity. In this deformity there is hyperextension of the proximal interphalangeal joint and flexion of the distal interphalangeal joint.
   b. Boutonniere deformity. In this deformity there is flexion at the proximal interphalangeal joint and hyperextension at the distal interphalangeal joint.

The causes of these deformities are complex and result from disease of the capsule, extensor hood/tendons and volar plate and interference with intrinsic muscle function.

Ganglion

Ganglions are a type of adventitious bursa with fibrous lining and containing clear but viscous liquid — almost a jelly. They may occur at many sites usually associated with joints or tendon sheaths and are quite harmless.

The reason for mentioning them in this section is that they are very common on the dorsum of the hand.

The cysts need not be removed but the surgeon is often persuaded to do so for reasons of pain and cosmesis. Because they may be multilocular and are closely applied to tendons etc. the surgeon is advised to remove them under general anaesthetic and tourniquet. It is advisable to warn the patient that they can recur after surgery.

Trigger thumb and trigger finger (stenosing tenovaginitis)

In the majority of cases this condition occurs without obvious cause. The fibrous flexor sheath thickens thus narrowing the lumen. The narrowed area frets the tendon creating a localized 'nodule'. As the nodule passes through the stenosed area a painful click or snap is felt and this is visible as 'triggering' of the digit. Sometimes the digit frankly locks in flexion and cannot be extended.

The student should know that a congenital type exists and that the presence of several triggering digits should make him or her think of the possibility of more generalized disease such as diabetes or rheumatoid arthritis.

Treatment is by slitting the stenosed sheath surgically.

Dupuytren's contracture

This is a disease of the palmar aponeurosis. The aetiology is unknown but there is an association with:

Family History
Alcoholism
Liver disease
Epilepsy

The disease occurs mainly in elderly males. The hands are usually affected but occasionally the feet as well. A vague association occurs rarely with Peyronies disease of the penis and retroperitoneal fibrosis.

The diagnosis is easy:
1. Nodules and puckerings of the palmar skin.
2. Contracture of metacarpophalangeal and proximal interphalangeal joints usually of the ulnar digits of the hand and visibly produced by tight palpable bands.
3. Some cases have 'knuckle pads' on the dorsum of the proximal interphalangeal joints.

Pathology

This is rather unsatisfying as histology shows merely hyperplasia of the palmar aponeurosis with increase in longitudinal collagen fibres.

Treatment
No treatment is required until contracture occurs. In general contractures of the proximal interphalangeal joint must be treated earlier than those of the metacarpophalangeal joint. The treatment is surgical with fasciotomy, local fasciectomy and rarely 'total' fasciectomy.

Miscellaneous conditions of the lower limb

THE HIP

In the first chapter the student will have learned how to examine the hip joint. Diseases of the hip present by pain, stiffness, instability or deformity. Above all the hip may be 'irritable'. This symptom indicates inflammation and should always be taken seriously. The pathology of the hip has been discussed in other chapters. One of the most likely conditions that a student may meet in his clinical examinations is osteoarthrosis of the hip. It is common in Europe and patients are frequently admitted to hospital for surgery and are hence 'available' for clinical examinations. Learn how to examine the hip joint and study the section on osteoarthrosis and its management.

Similarly there are several important conditions of the hip in childhood which are popular with examiners. These are discussed under the heading of 'Paediatric Orthopaedics'. Learn about these conditions. Remember also these points:

1. The 'hip' may be part of the symptom complex of back—buttock—leg pain.

2. Hip joint pain is often referred to the thigh and to the knee especially in children.

3. Instability of the hip presents with an instability gait. Think of 'power-fulcrum-levers' to explain such a gait.

4. The commonest deformities of the hip are fixed flexion, adduction and external rotation, but patients are more likely to complain of shortening.

5. Osteoarthrosis tends to present with pain, stiffness and loss of function. Inflammatory arthritides of the hip tend to present with 'irritability', i.e. acute pain and voluntary resistance to any movement, particularly internal rotation.

Coxa vara

This is a condition where the normal neck–shaft angle of the femur becomes more acute than normal. It may be congenital, follow slipped upper femoral epiphysis, result from malunion of a fracture or bone softening due to local or generalized bone disease. The point is that coxa vara may result in shortening and an instability limp. (In this case due to approximation of the origin to the insertion of the powerful hip abductors 'power and levers!')

Trochanteric bursitis

Although inflammation of the trochanteric bursa may occasionally be tuberculous (in those countries where the disease is often seen), the more usual cause is non-specific inflammation. Typically pain is felt at the greater trochanter and radiates down the ilio-tibial band. Local tenderness is usual. Treatment varies from the use of anti-inflammatory drugs and physiotherapy to local steroid injection.

Intra-abdominal, retroperitoneal and pelvic infection

Pain in the hip and deformity caused by muscle spasm may occasionally arise from infection at these sites. Think of this when no other explanation for pain and spasm can be found in the hip. Examine the abdomen and perform a rectal examination.

THE KNEE JOINT

In orthopaedic pathology 'things tend to happen around the knee joint'. For example acute osteitis, bone tumours and exostoses are common near the knee. Osteoarthritis and the inflammatory arthritides affect the knee. Loose bodies commonly present here and it is the site of osteochondritis dissecans and pathological ossification.

The knee is probably also the commonest site for serious sporting injuries and other trauma. Its specialized ligaments and menisci are vulnerable and give rise to a number of mechanical disorders.

The classic symptoms of mechanical disorders of the knee are pain, swelling, locking and giving way.

Ligament injuries to the knee —— see page 99.

Tears of the menisci — see page 103.

Other disorders of menisci
Note that whereas meniscal tears are 5–6 times commoner on the medial side of the knee, other meniscal lesions are much commoner on the lateral side.

Cysts of the menisci
These cysts are ganglion-like cystic cavities occuring in a dense proliferation of fibrous tissue at the outer margin of a meniscus. They form a 'lump' in the joint line which usually feels firm and not cystic. The lump may fluctuate in size and in the severity of symptoms.

Clinical features
There is a history of persisting low-grade pain associated with a 'lump' in the joint line usually of lateral meniscus. The 'lump' is usually tender on firm pressure. It is best felt when the knee is slightly flexed and compared in this position with the normal side.

Treatment
If symptoms justify interference then meniscectomy is the treatment of choice.

Discoid lateral meniscus
This is a congenital deformity of the meniscus due to persistence of the embryonic shape, i.e. a 'disc' of meniscus and not a semi-lunar shaped structure persists.

   The condition presents usually in childhood and adolescence with pain, giving way and locking of the knee. Often a history of a loud 'clunking' of the knee during movements is given by the patient.

   Despite the surgeon's reluctance to remove menisci in young people, symptoms may justify arthroscopy and subsequent meniscectomy if the diagnosis is confirmed.

Recurrent dislocation of the patella
The initial dislocation is caused usually by trauma but there is often an underlying abnormality which predisposes the patella to this dislocation — hence the trauma may be slight.

   Typically the patellae are small or high, the lateral

condyle underdeveloped or the knee valgus in shape. Females are much more prone to this condition than males.

Clinical features
During some sporting or other activity involving flexion and extension of the knee while weight bearing, the patella dislocates laterally and appears to be 'standing on its edge'. It may reduce spontaneously or require reduction under anaesthesia. A haemarthrosis follows and there is tenderness over the medial retinaculum — which must tear to allow lateral dislocation. A single dislocation requires only immobilization in a plaster cylinder followed by physiotherapy.

Recurrent dislocation should cause the doctor to look for predisposing causes. If the dislocations are frequent there may well be quadriceps wasting and the physical sign of patellar 'apprehension'. The patient feels pain and a sensation of impending dislocation when the patella is forcibly pushed laterally during flexion and extension of the knee.

Troublesome recurrent dislocations require surgery. The principles are that a lateral soft tissue release should be performed with or without transposition of the tibial tuberosity to a more medial position, thus straightening the line of pull of the quadriceps muscles, and weakening their lateral pull.

Rupture of the quadriceps mechanism
The extensor mechanism of the knee is often torn in association with fracture of the patella. However, it also occurs at the site of the attachment of the quadriceps tendon to the patella or less commonly through the patellar ligament itself. This injury usually occurs in middle life or later. The patient is unable to lift the leg with the knee extended. Tenderness and a palpable 'gap' can be felt at the rupture site. Surgical repair is usually required.

Chondromalacia patellae
This is a troublesome and ill understood condition of adolescents and young adults in which degenerative changes occur on the articular surface of the patella resulting in fibrillation, roughening and sometimes frank ulceration of the

articular cartilage. It is usually self limiting and does not usually progress directly to osteoarthrosis in the patello-femoral compartment.

Clinical features
The patient complains of an aching pain in the knee usually anterior but typically aggravated by descending stairs or sitting for prolonged periods with the knees flexed.

Sometimes an effusion is present but more commonly there is only tenderness at the margins of the patella (displace it and palpate deeply) or on 'rubbing' the patella firmly across the underlying femur. Radiographs are usually normal.

Treatment should be conservative. (Remember the majority of your patients will get better spontaneously.) A variety of treatments are used with variable success. Static quadriceps exercises and short-wave diathermy is a widely practised regime. In severe and recalcitrant cases surgery is (reluctantly) advised. A variety of surgical procedures is practised indicating the uncertainty of the results of any one procedure. It is not within the scope of this book to go into further detail concerning these procedures.

Cysts and bursae around the knee

Bursae are common around the knee. The prepatellar bursa (housemaid's knee) and the infrapatellar bursa (clergyman's knee) are both the result of the repeated trauma of prolonged and repeated kneeling. The bursae are clearly visible and palpable as cystic swellings. The knee joint itself is normal.

Repeated aspiration may cure the condition but sometimes surgical excision is required.

Cysts in the popliteal fossa are quite common.

The Baker's cyst is a soft diffuse swelling formed by bulging and herniation of the synovium. This popular eponym (popular with examiners!) is often misused. The important point is that a true 'Baker's cyst' is secondary to other pathology of the knee, e.g. osteoarthrosis or inflammatory arthritis. This pathology is usually apparent clinically.

The semimembranosus bursa occurs between the semimembranosus tendon and deeper structures. It forms a cyst which may be soft or tense in the medial side of the popliteal fossa. This is usually seen in children and young adults.

These popliteal cysts do not always require active treatment. Surgery should be reserved for those cases where diagnosis is in doubt or the cyst becomes tense and painful.

Note that popliteal cysts are difficult to feel with the knee flexed and easier to feel with the patient standing. Examination from behind will then permit the clinician to compare the popliteal fossa with that of the other side.

THE CALF AND SHIN

Calf pain

Pain in the calf may be referred from the spine. If swelling and tenderness are present think of the possibility of ruptures of popliteal cysts, or gastrocnemius tears or of deep vein thrombosis. Denervated muscle is said to be tender.

Pain in the shin may occur due to overexertion, stress fracture or anterior tibial compartment syndrome. Always take radiographs to exclude other pathology. A careful history may lead the clinician to suspect one of these conditions.

Intermittent claudication

This is a pain in the leg, particularly the calf, which occurs on exercise and disappears as soon as the exercise discontinues. It is nearly always due to relative ischaemia and indicates peripheral vascular disease. A careful history and examination of pedal pulses will usually allow correct diagnosis. There may be other evidence of peripheral ischaemia.

Remember also that spinal pathology may give rise to claudication-like symptoms occasionally.

Paratendonitis and rupture of the tendo-achilles

Pain in the lower calf and calcaneal tendon is often due to a paratendonitis probably the result of degenerative changes in the tendon.

Pain, tenderness and local swelling are usually present. Treatment is by rest and non-steroidal anti-inflammatory drugs. Some patients are helped by a small temporary heel raise to the shoe.

The condition predisposes the patient to rupture of the tendo-Achilles but many cases of the rupture have no previous relevant history.

Rupture of the tendo-Achilles usually takes place during heavy exercise. The patient feels pain and feels 'something go' or a sense of 'being kicked at the back of the ankle'. The difficulty in diagnosis is that the patient can walk with a limp and local haemorrhage and swelling may obscure the 'gap' in the tendon.

The condition is easy to miss. Always palpate the tendo-Achilles carefully after injuries to 'the ankle'. The patient cannot stand on tiptoe. If the patient is asked to kneel with his feet over the edge of the couch it may be noticed that squeezing of the calves will fail to produce ankle flexion on the affected side. Note that some active flexion can be performed by the long flexors of the toes — and beware!

The rupture is nearly always complete. Surgical repair is preferred by most surgeons but others prefer to immobilize the leg in an equinus plaster for eight weeks.

PAIN IN THE ANKLE

The ankle suffers at times from the usual cross section of arthritides and frequently from trauma.

The secret of examination of the ankle and foot is to control the heel with one hand during examination and to palpate the ankle and foot with the other.

Flexion and extension of the foot and heel together is then pure ankle movement.

Inversion and eversion of the foot and heel together is then mainly subtalar joint movement.

Immobilization of the heel and rotation at the forefoot then tests the midfoot joints.

The ankle is a superficial joint with well-recognized bony points that can be inspected and palpated in the usual way.

Chronic 'sprain' and recurrent subluxation of the ankle
This condition usually arises in a patient who has a history of a previous acute 'sprain'.

The patient gives a history of repeated episodes of 'going over' (i.e. inversion) of the ankle which 'gives way' and is followed by pain and swelling lasting a few days or weeks.

Examination close to the time of the injury will show local tenderness, swelling and bruising but examination at a later date often offers little to find. Some local tenderness over the anterior part of the lateral ligament of the ankle is usually present.

Radiographs should be taken in the standard positions and also of both ankles with the feet forced into inversion. These 'strain' views may show opening of the joint on the lateral side (subluxation of the diseased ankle compared with the normal side. If frank subluxation is present and episodes frequent then a surgical reconstruction of the lateral ligament may be indicated. Most cases, however, are not as severe as this and simple physiotherapy to strengthen inversion and eversion may be adequate to relieve the condition. 'Floating out' and raising the outer edge of the heel of the shoe may also be tried.

PAIN IN THE FOOT

Adult flat foot and foot strain

The subject of flat foot has been discussed in the section entitled 'Paediatric Orthopaedics'. Flat feet are not necessarily bad feet but often in middle age, patients with flat feet may complain of pain under the longitudinal arch. This may be helped by longitudinal arch insoles. Some surgeons place great faith in physiotherapy with exercises and faradic stimulation of muscles but this is time consuming and of doubtful value.

Foot strain may also be caused by prolonged standing, e.g. change of job, prolonged marching etc.

These conditions are difficult to distinguish from and indeed may merge into osteoarthrosis of the mid foot joints. This is usually apparent clinically and radiologically. Again arch supports may be of assistance. Rarely is surgery required.

Peroneal spastic flat foot is a condition where disease in the subtalar joint results in pains, eversion of the hindfoot and pronation of the forefoot associated with visible spasm of the peroneal muscles. The importance is that the disease in the subtalar joint must be identified and treated.

'March' fracture

This is a stress fracture of a metatarsal bone, usually the second or third. It is associated with prolonged and perhaps unaccustomed exercise. Think of this condition when there is a good history and there is localized tenderness and 'puffiness' of the dorsum of the forefoot. Radiographs may not show the stress fracture initially but later films will show a little callus as the fracture heals. Rest or a period of immobilization in a plaster cast will cure the condition.

Pain in the heel

What the patient means by the 'heel' is not necessarily the same as you understand. Does the patient mean:

Under the heel? — bruised heel
— plantar fasciitis
— os calcis pathology

At the back of the heel? — calcaneal paratendonitis
— postcalcaneal bursitis
— calcaneal 'bumps'
— calcaneal apophysitis (children).

Vaguely in the hindfoot? — Arthritis of the ankle or subtalar joint.
— tenosynovitis of tibialis posterior tendon

Obtain this history carefully and then examine the ankle, the subtalar joints, the calcaneum and the adjacent tendons. If this regime is followed the diagnosis will usually become apparent.

Postcalcaneal bursitis and calcaneal 'bumps'

These are related conditions usually found in young girls. The os calcis is often high and prominent posteriorly and laterally with a 'bump' and a tender bursa between the 'bump' and the skin. Surgical excision of bursa and 'bump' may be required in troublesome cases.

Planter fasciitis

This is an inflammatory disease of uncertain origin

affecting the attachment of the plantar fascia to the medial calcaneal tubercle. A few cases may be associated with a more generalized disease, e.g. Reiter's syndrome.

The history is diagnostic. The patient, usually a middle-aged woman, complains of pain 'under the heel'. The pain is worse on standing after a period of rest, e.g. on first arising in the morning, and eases off with walking about.

Examination is precise. Firm pressure on the medial calcaneal tubercle reproduces the pain. The patient is often impressed with the experienced clinician's ability to place his or her finger 'exactly on the spot'.

Radiographs may show a calcaneal spur but this is of doubtful relevance. The main value of the radiographs is to exclude pathology in the os calcis.

Treatment is by providing a soft heel pad and prescribing a powerful non-steroidal anti-inflammatory drug. Some clinicians use local steroid injections but these are painful and often not appreciated by the patient!

Metatarsalgia (pain in the forefoot)

This is usually pain under the metatarsal heads ('under the tread'). Occasionally the pain is more widely felt in the forefoot. The majority of cases arise in middle-aged ladies who have a dropped transverse arch and excess weight carrying on the 2nd and 3rd metatarsal heads. This is often associated with broadening of the forefoot and hallux valgus. Examination of the sole shows the callosities associated with excess weight bearing. The condition is relieved by provision of a weight relieving insole. Occasionally surgical 'elevation' of the affected metatarsal head by osteotomy of the relevant metatarsal bone may be required.

A much rarer cause is March fracture (vide supra).

Occasionally a plantar digital neuroma may be responsible (Morton's metatarsalgia). This is a fibrous thickening of a digital nerve probably due to chronic trauma. It is usually found in the cleft between the 3rd and 4th toes just distal to the relevant metatarsal heads. The condition occurs typically in middle-aged women. Sometimes a history of pain radiating to the relevant toes may be elicited. Lateral pressure (squeezing) the forefoot may produce a painful click.

The diagnosis is difficult to distinguish from metatarsalgia of other causes. Exploration may be indicated if an appropriate weight-relieving insole does not relieve the symptoms. If the neuroma is found it should be excised.

Plantar warts, corns and callosities
The majority of local thickenings of the skin of the foot occur as a result of excess local pressure, e.g. dropped transverse arch or toe deformity.

Sometimes a plantar wart may be responsbile. This has the appearance of an ingrowing wart with thickened skin around it. Classically severe pain is produced on squeezing it from side to side rather than pressure applied to its surface. Small plantar warts may be difficult to distinguish from 'tintack' corns.

TOE DEFORMITIES

Hallux valgus and bunions
This is a common condition in females. The great toe drifts laterally exposing the first metatarsal head and thus creating a medial 'bump' or 'bunion' which becomes covered with a bursa and thickened skin (Fig. 48). As the toe drifts laterally it becomes less efficient and the second and third metatarsal

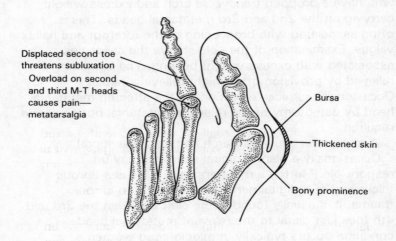

Displaced second toe threatens subluxation

Overload on second and third M-T heads causes pain— metatarsalgia

Bursa

Thickened skin

Bony prominence

Fig. 48 The story of neglected Hallux valgus—bunion, subluxation of the second metatarsophalangeal joint and metatarsalgia.

heads bear more weight. This may lead to concurrent metatarsalgia.

It is used to be thought that tight shoewear was responsible for this condition but this is probably untrue. The inherited foot shape, torsional shape of the legs, forefoot pronation etc. probably predispose the foot to this condition in the majority of cases. Some are due to excess broadening of the forefoot (metatarsus primus varus). Whatever the underlying cause the tight shoewear is thus merely an aggravating factor.

It is important during history taking to elicit exactly what is bothering the patient. If pain is present find out whether it is the bunion itself or metatarsalgia which is causing the pain. Some patients are worried about the appearance, and some worried because they have difficulty in purchasing comfortable (and fashionable) shoes.

Treatment should not be regarded as an 'automatic' decision. Mild cases are probably best advised against surgery and helped with advice concerning shoewear, footcare etc. Those with metatarsalgia should be treated with extreme caution. If symptoms are severe surgery is indicated, but beware! these operations have a bad reputation because patients expect too much too soon! In fact, well-chosen surgery is usually very successful. The well-known Keller's operation (an excision arthroplasty) is effective in older patients but those with metatarsalgia should be advised to undergo a first metatarsal corrective osteotomy or sometimes arthrodesis of the first metatarsophalangeal joint.

Hammer toe and claw toes

A hammer toe is a toe (usually the second) with a fixed flexion deformity of the proximal interphalangeal joint usually with extension of the distal joint and a painful overlying callosity. Surgical correction and fusion of the joint is a reliable procedure.

In claw toes, both interphalangeal joints are flexed but usually correctable and multiple callosities occur. Often these toes are associated with excess weight bearing on the metatarsal heads. Conservative treatment should be preferred but in severe cases surgical fusion of the appropriate joints may be performed.

Hallux rigidus

This is an osteoarthrosis of the first metatarsophalangeal joint but often occurring at a much younger age than would be generally expected. It occurs commonly in men. The aetiology is uncertain.

The joint is stiff and painful and often enlarged by osteophytes.

Radiographs show the features of osteoarthrosis.

Conservative treatment with metatarsal bars (rocker bars) may help some cases. If the condition is severe the joint must either be excised (excision arthroplasty) or fused (arthrodesis).

Ingrowing toenail and onychogryposis

Everybody is aware of ingrowing toenails as they are a familiar part of human experience.

The corner·and edge of the nail of the great toe digs into the skin and causes pain. Secondary infection commonly occurs with pain, infected granulation and discharge. Some of the nails are manifestly deformed with thickening and increased curvature. Others are large and flat and seemingly of good shape. Improper cutting of toenails contributes to the deformity and often provokes infection.

There is a considerable volume of writing on this subject and opinions differ. The author suggests the following regime.
1. If not infected the nail should be treated conservatively. It should be allowed to grow and cut square at the end. Tangential filing helps to weaken the nail and prevent 'digging in' at the corners. If the patient can be persuaded to pack small rolls of cotton wool under the corners of the nail—so much the better.
2. If pain is excessive or infection established it is preferable to avulse the nail on the first occasion. The patient can then attempt to treat the new nail conservatively as above.
3. If recurrent problems occur, then surgical or chemical ablation of the nail bed to prevent further nail growth is simple and effective. The author sees little advantage in partial excision of the nail and nail bed but this procedure is widely practised.

Onchogryposis is a horn-like thickening and deformity of

the great toenail usually occurring in the elderly. If chiropody cannot control the nail, then surgical ablation of the nail bed should be performed.

The great toenail is often deformed as a result of injury, may be lifted by subungual exostoses and infected with fungal infections. Occasionally subungual melanomata occur.

THE SIGNIFICANCE OF DIABETES MELLITUS AND PERIPHERAL VASCULAR DISEASE IN SURGICAL CONDITIONS OF THE FOOT.

It is imperative that the peripheral pulses should be examined in every case where surgery to the lower limb is contemplated. In peripheral vascular disease surgery may be followed by failure to heal, sepsis and even frank gangrene. Beware!

Similarly patients who have toe deformities, corns, ulcerated callosities etc. and who also have peripheral vascular disease must be treated with extreme care. Such minor lesions may precipitate ulceration and gangrene. Such patients should be instructed in the regular care of their feet.

The diabetic foot

Diabetic patients are also at risk from ulceration and sepsis arising in minor lesions of the toes. Elderly diabetics may simply have atherosclerosis, but younger diabetics have a peripheral small vessel arteriopathy associated with their disease. They are thus vulnerable to infection, ulceration and local gangrene.

The reasons for this are:
1. Arteriopathy of small vessels.
2. Raised blood sugar and possibly abnormalities of immune response encourage infections.
3. Neuropathy:
    a. diminished pain sensation
    b. toe deformities due to intrinsic muscle weakness
    c. altered vascular response to inflammation

The basic principles of management of the diabetic foot are as follows:
1. Control the diabetes.

2. Admit the patient, rest and elevate the foot.
3. Antibiotics where indicated.
4. If local gangrene occurs then it should be excised locally. Surgery should be conservative.

Index